PRINCIPLES FOR
FIRST AID
FOR THE INJURED

PRINCIPLES FOR FIRST AID FOR THE INJURED

THIRD EDITION

H. PROCTOR, MB, BS, FRCSE
Lately Orthopaedic Surgeon, Birmingham Accident Hospital

P. S. LONDON, MBE, CStJ, MB, BS, FRCS
Surgeon, Birmingham Accident Hospital

BUTTERWORTHS
LONDON - BOSTON
Sydney - Wellington - Durban - Toronto

The Butterworth Group

United Kingdom	**Butterworth & Co (Publishers) Ltd**
London	88 Kingsway, WC2B 6AB
Australia	**Butterworths Pty Ltd**
Sydney	586 Pacific Highway, Chatswood, NSW 2067
	Also at Melbourne, Brisbane, Adelaide and Perth
South Africa	**Butterworth & Co (South Africa) (Pty) Ltd**
Durban	152–154 Gale Street
New Zealand	**Butterworths of New Zealand Ltd**
Wellington	26–28 Waring Taylor Street, 1
Canada	**Butterworth & Co (Canada) Ltd**
Toronto	2265 Midland Avenue, Scarborough, Ontario, M1P 4S1
USA	**Butterworth (Publishers) Inc**
Boston	19 Cummings Park, Woburn, Mass. 01801

First Published 1962

Reprinted 1964

Second Edition 1968

Third Edition 1977

ISBN 0 407 36441 2

© Butterworth & Co (Publishers) Ltd 1977

Library of Congress Cataloging in Publication Data

Proctor, Henry, British surgeon.
   Principles for first aid for the injured.

   Bibliography: p
   Includes index.
   1. First aid in illness and injury. I. London,
Peter Stanford, joint author. II. Title. [DNLM:
1. First aid. WA292 P964p]
RC87.P8 1976 614.8'8 76-40483
ISBN 0-407-36441-2

Typeset by Butterworths Litho Preparation Department

Made and printed in Great Britain by Butler & Tanner Ltd, London and Frome

For indeed it is one of the lessons of the history of science that each age steps on the shoulders of the ages which have gone before. The value of each age is not its own, but is in part, in large part, a debt to its forerunners. And this age of ours, if, like its predecessors, it can boast something of which it is proud, would, could it read the future, doubtless find much also of which it would be ashamed.

SIR MICHAEL FOSTER

CONTENTS

PREFACE TO
THE THIRD EDITION

When dealing with principles there is the advantage that they change little or not at all, and certainly much less than the practices that are derived from them. Nevertheless, when planning a new edition authors will ask themselves whether the literary garment they are tending will bear a few more tucks here, some letting out there and an assortment of patches, or whether the time has come to discard the original pattern and devise a new one.

In First Aid there is much that is unchanging—for example the general nature of the accidents that are occurring in ever-increasing numbers and the harmful effects they have on the human body. The forces to which man subjects himself or is subjected to have long since passed the point at which even the most heroic measures can bring about survival but there have been remarkable advances in the field of resuscitation, most notably in the war in Vietnam, that have taken what is possible far beyond what was hardly conceivable as recently as 10 years ago. These advances have been less in the techniques of diagnosis and treatment than in making existing techniques available earlier and earlier after injury, and applying them with greater energy and a lavish abundance of men and material.

For these reasons, the general pattern of the book has been retained, with appropriate deletions and additions, but a new chapter has been prepared to give an account of trends in First Aid and other sorts of emergency care, trends that owe something to the humane attitudes that are not extinguished by even the most barbaric cruelties of war. With this chapter is another new feature—a list of books and articles for further reading. The greatest difficulty was to decide how few titles and authors to quote; our choice was made with general readers in mind in the belief that specialists such as accident and emergency surgeons would have means of extending their reading that some of their comrades in service would not.

Birmingham   H.P.
                                                                P.S.L.

PREFACE TO
THE SECOND EDITION

Since the first edition of this book there have been striking changes in the joint manual of the voluntary First Aid societies and a working party has recommended a much higher standard of training for ambulance crews, for which term 'Ambulance Aid' is being preferred in some quarters to 'First Aid'. The changes concerned are in the matters of detail and range; they do not depend upon changes in the principles upon which rest the properly varied practices of, for example, boy scouts, uniformed members of the voluntary First Aid societies, ambulance crews, miners, mountain rescue parties, nurses and doctors when they carry out the first useful treatment of someone who has suffered injury or sudden illness.

The changes in this edition reflect changes in knowledge, particularly of drowning and of exposure, and the introduction of the principle of pneumatic support for injured limbs. In the revised chapters dealing with shock and injury and we have tried to emphasize that shock is a term that should not be applied indiscriminately and thoughtlessly to practically all victims of injury but restricted to those changes that injury causes in the pattern of circulation and that are mostly dependent upon diminishing blood volume. In spite of the confusing range of senses in which the word shock is used and the belief that its erasure from the medical vocabulary would in the long term make for clarity we have retained the word because it is conveniently brief and because it can be defined for our purpose.

In closing this Preface we wish to acknowledge our indebtedness to those many persons at all levels of emergency services and First Aid and allied movements that have given us the benefit of their opinions, advice and experience.

Birmingham   H.P.
                                                           P.S.L.

PREFACE TO
THE FIRST EDITION

This is not just another book about First Aid but is intended as an exposition of modern ideas and practices in the care of the injured and of the principles upon which they are based. The idea of the book was conceived by the late Ruscoe Clarke, whose experience of forward surgery during World War II, followed by 12 years at the Birmingham Accident Hospital, gave him an excellent appreciation of the needs of injured persons. His breadth of vision and his sure grasp of essentials led him to the conclusion that while these needs were widely acknowledged at humanitarian level their interpretation in practice lacked precision. This precision depended upon accurate knowledge of the advances that he outstandingly among others had helped to make in applying scientific methods to the treatment of injuries of all kinds. From the commanding position that his experience allowed him he was able to survey the whole field of the care of the injured and to recognize that he and his kind must accept the responsibility of pointing out deficiencies with the constructive type of criticism that enabled them to be made good.

His intense and unflagging interest in people as individuals directed his thoughts and activities towards the preliminary care of those who had suffered injury. He devoted much time to the subject of First Aid and received increasing calls for advice and assistance as a lecturer, writer and examiner. His main researches since 1947 have done much to elucidate the nature and treatment of shock and haemorrhage, and to emphasize the need to recognize promptly that treatment may have to be immediate if lives are to be saved and recovery facilitated. The over-riding necessity is to avoid the delay that can readily jeopardize survival and curtail the successful application of advances in resuscitation, surgery and anaesthesia to the repair of injuries. This new emphasis on urgency has entailed acknowledging that the delay inherent in some traditional First Aid can at times exert an unfavourable influence on the effects of injury, especially serious injury.

His purpose in preparing this book was to offer the fruits of rich experience to those responsible for teaching and organizing in the field

xiii

of First Aid and kindred activities. He sought to provide them with a sound foundation for a system of early care that could be applied with benefit by those without special skill or training: it had above all to be a logical precursor to the appropriate medical treatment. In this he was following the example of the originator of First Aid—Esmarch. He intended the book for medical men in the First Aid movement and for senior, non-medical teachers and practitioners in this field. It was to provide them with a synoptic and reasoned view of the diagnosis and treatment of injuries and to show how modern ideas and practices should guide the practice and teaching of First Aid, particularly in eliminating methods that have been, and may yet be, invalidated by the advance of ideas.

At the time of his death in the summer of 1959 Mr. Clarke had not proceeded beyond a draft of the outline of the book, which was to have been a joint work by himself and the senior of the present authors. Far from weakening this project, the death of its originator provided a stimulus for its fulfilment and the original plan has been retained with few modifications.

The term First Aid has been used throughout and it will be seen that it has been allowed two senses. In the first it means the practice approved by the voluntary aid societies; in the second it reverts to its original meaning of preliminary treatment. While we have used the form with capital letters we have sought by indiscriminate use of the two senses to emphasize our belief that there should be but one meaning of these two words.

The field covered is much greater than that customarily allowed to First Aid. First, new sorts and severities of injuries are now increasingly occurring and they pose new problems in diagnosis and treatment. Secondly, definitive treatment of severe injuries is more effective and more often successful than before—provided there is a living person to treat. Thirdly, in some conditions definitive treatment may be long delayed and preliminary treatment may necessarily be something more than makeshift patching up and prompt despatch to hospital.

Birmingham   H.P.
P.S.L.

1

INTRODUCTION

The exponents of First Aid are essentially enthusiastic people who have also a wish to be of service and assistance to their fellows in time of trouble. Enthusiasm is fostered, recruiting assisted and proficiency developed by lectures, demonstrations and, above all, by competitions and awards. These admirable and necessary activities have understandably concentrated on the more readily practicable parts of First Aid, which are as a result carried out competently when called for. Subtler but important aspects, such as changes in colour, variations in tone, obliteration of pulses and progressive swelling of limbs cannot be reproduced and, being in consequence less familiar to First Aiders, may escape their attention or lead perhaps to lost opportunities. The needs of an unconscious person, for example, may be more urgent than those of a person with an obvious wound or fracture. Valuable though casualty simulation can be, unless it is used with proper understanding it may seem to emphasize practical skill rather than judgment and sound decision.

As medical knowledge and practice advances the type of First Aid that can usefully be applied necessarily changes.

The most numerous injuries are of small size and carry little risk to limb or life; changes in First Aid have been in matters of detail. Fashions change but the basic treatment for a wound is to cover it with a suitable dressing. With fractures, First Aid is essentially a matter of making the part comfortable and preventing further damage. The use of a splint is only one way of doing this and the concept of splintage might be better replaced by the practice of providing comfortable support.

THE ACCIDENT PROBLEM IN GREAT BRITAIN

Although there can be few First Aiders outside the organized rescue services that have had any experience of serious injury, the fact that some 20,000 lives and many times more limbs are endangered each year makes it highly desirable that as many as possible of the population should have some knowledge of what to do. As well as the dramatic effect of injury there are the unnumbered throngs of minor casualties, and those taken suddenly ill are as much in need of knowledgeable attention as are the injured.

The figures in Table 1.1 indicate the current size of the problem, which has been growing year by year. It will be noted that whereas the number of discharges after admission for all causes rose by one-third in 10 years, the corresponding figure for injuries rose by one-half. First Aid, First Aiders, and their teachers need to keep pace with the advances in both numbers and standards of emergency treatment.

TABLE 1.1
Accidents in England and Wales

Deaths in 1973 from accidents

On the roads	6,890
In homes	6,158
At work	692
Burns and scalds	627
Total	16,652

Persons injured by road accidents in 1973

Seriously	82,030*
Slightly	235,696

*Each caused at least 3 days' absence from work.

Table 1.2 gives some idea of the cost to the nation of industrial injuries and their effects. Apparently trivial injuries can lead to prolonged absence from work if they are not properly diagnosed and treated.

TABLE 1.2
Industrial injuries in England and Wales in 1973

Killed at work	692
Notifiable accidents	256,930*

*Each caused at least 3 days' absence from work.

PROGRESS IN TEACHING FIRST AID

Some of what has been said may seem to lay the responsibility for shortcomings in present-day First Aid upon the First Aid movement itself, but fundamentally the lag of First Aid behind the most up-to-date treatment of the injured is the result of a lack of an holistic approach to their care. What is needed is a return to a broad outlook so that First Aid and hospital treatment shall be properly co-ordinated.

It is not sufficient to expect the medical men in First Aid organizations to keep abreast of advances, for most of them have either retired from active medical practice or are engaged in the public health service or general practice, which gives them neither time nor opportunity to keep in touch with other fields of medicine. Those doctors who devote their time to the treatment of injuries must be prepared to play their part in the development of First Aid to keep it in step with relevant changes in medical and surgical ideas and practice. This is not to suggest that hospital and other suitably experienced doctors should take it upon themselves to lay down the rules and drill for First Aid, but that they should pass on the knowledge upon which the rules and drills should be based.

The problems that arise in the training of large numbers of people contrast strikingly with the direction and supervision of trained hospital staffs. Enthusiasm and a sense of service are outstanding features throughout the First Aid movement but they are not universally matched by intelligence or education. Modern methods of treating injuries, especially serious injuries, require careful attention to detail and perhaps frequent and rapid changes to keep pace with the changes in the condition of the person under treatment. Such flexibility cannot be extended outside hospital, and before a new type of treatment can be offered to the First Aid movement to be included in its training it must be adapted so as to be generally and safely applicable to a variety of conditions that may be distinguishable only by the expert in his hospital with all sorts of diagnostic and therapeutic assistance at his beck and call. Frills must be eliminated, complexity must give way to simplicity in both diagnosis and treatment so that the objective—the useful preliminary care of the injured person—shall be attainable in any foreseeable emergency. The most important step is to inculcate a clear appreciation of the order of priority in treatment; to teach dogmatically the most urgent conditions, how they are to be recognized (which may mean looking specially for them) and how they should be treated. Less serious conditions may also require treatment, but in some circumstances they may have to be passed over for the sake of avoiding delay that might prove fatal. A person dead of respiratory obstruction will have derived no benefit from skilfully applied dressings and splints.

There is, therefore, need for translating definitive needs into terms and practices generally and usefully applicable as First Aid. The translation can be achieved only by the close association of hospital doctors who care for the injured and the directing members of the First Aid movement. Given this it should be possible to keep First Aid well up-to-date. It may be objected that this would lead to frequent changes in First Aid practice and that the frequent issue of revised manuals would sow confusion in the minds of many First Aiders. This objection is not likely to be serious in practice because advances take place fairly slowly as a rule, and by using appropriate amendments and supplements it would rarely be necessary to revise successive editions of First Aid manuals drastically. It may be doubted whether serious confusion would arise, because First Aiders are notably anxious to be up-to-date. However proud they may be of past achievements, they can usually be relied upon to accept and adopt new methods with enthusiasm, especially if the need for changes be made clear to them.

By keeping abreast of advances through the close co-operation of doctors with the necessary time, interest and knowledge, First Aiders can be encouraged to feel, as indeed they are, important members of the greater medical team for the care of the injured. Though disappointed by the excision of outmoded methods of treatment in which they had become expert and taken a just pride, they could be consoled by a recognition that their loss has been the patient's gain. Nor is it all loss, because with injuries of the chest and head it has been shown that active treatment of the right kind can do much to enable patients to reach hospital alive and with a good prospect of recovery. First Aid has a new and increased scope here. There is also the need for careful observation at the scene of the accident and of the patient's condition and progress. The reports that can sometimes be given may be of decisive importance to the hospital doctors, who in their turn must be made aware of the need to seek all the information they can from those who have information to impart.

In addition to general First Aid as at present taught and practised, appropriately modified First Aid should be available to individuals and teams who have frequent experience of accidents. As examples, there are ambulance crews and mine and other rescue services. The practical experience gained by these would serve as a sound foundation for teaching special methods appropriate to the types of accidents they would be likely to encounter. Because of their familiarity with injuries, such persons would be more likely to have a degree of judgment that would enable them to apply more detailed, more flexible and more advanced methods of treatment with success. Members of rescue teams are, moreover, likely to be carefully picked and therefore to be more reliable than the man in the street who has 'done a bit of First Aid'.

In recent years new standards of training have been introduced in the ambulance services and although the syllabus has gone far beyond what used to be thought of as First Aid, the same principles exist and deserve to be emphasized as such. Also, doctors have become increasingly eager to provide the First (medical) Aid available to the victims of road accidents. Theris is a special skill and experience but it is still recognizably derived from what is best in 'ordinary' First Aid.

The need is for continual review of First Aid in the light of scientific and other advances in hospital treatment and close co-operation between those who make the advances, those who translate them into First Aid, those who teach them and those who learn and do. Given this, the place and importance of First Aid is assured for as long as man is susceptible to injury.

2

PRINCIPLES OF TREATMENT

The essential purpose of First Aid is to provide such care as will benefit the patient preparatory to definitive treatment. The key word is 'benefit', because whether or not good will be done to the injured person will depend not upon the treatment given but upon the usefulness of that treatment in the particular circumstances. Treatment beneficial to a broken leg as the only injury in a person who has to travel far to hospital may be detrimental if that same person is also severely injured in the chest, an ambulance is waiting and the hospital is but a few minutes away. Treatment that can be provided is not necessarily treatment that should be provided, no matter how skilfully carried out nor how ingeniously devised.

The most important need is to save life. Compared with this, it is of secondary importance to facilitate definitive treatment. Desperate emergencies are not frequent in the experience of the man in the street in civil life in peace time. Not having had occasion to deal with anything so dramatic, should he be called upon to do so, suddenly and without preparation, he may be bewildered by the number and severity of the injuries before him and have difficulty in recognizing the relative urgency of the several injuries.

GENERAL CONSIDERATIONS

Life may be endangered by the effects of the injuries or by their causes. Among the outstanding effects of injury are severe external bleeding and embarrassment of respiration by obstruction of the air passages or damage to the chest. Both can kill very rapidly and both are usually responsive to First Aid. Other rapidly fatal conditions are beyond the scope of First Aid and need not be considered. The causes of injury that need urgent attention are noxious fumes and

6

gases, electricity, burning, the risk of explosion or flood and collapse of a nearby building, vehicle or other structure.

First Aid intended to facilitate definitive treatment of injuries comprises the dressing of wounds and arrest of less severe bleeding; the alignment, when necessary, and the support of broken limbs or spine; the promotion of comfort with pads or pillows, and protection from an unfavourable environment. This last will often mean controlling the attentions of bystanders and preventing well-meaning meddling or officious interference. The official recommendation that nuisances be disposed of by a judicious choice of errands and other activities that will take them away from the scene of the accident is admirable. On the other hand, it may be possible to press into service mildly injured persons either as active assistants or as passive observers. Apart from the possible value of their efforts, the fact that they are occupied by something other than their own misfortunes relieves the First Aider of some of his burden and allows him to concentrate his activities where they will be most beneficial.

When there are several casualties, the urge to treat the first one encountered must often be resisted until the general conditions have been appraised and the most urgent needs decided. This may require an agonizing choice between dealing with the dying and attending to others whose conditions can be improved by First Aid. The choice has to be made by those on the spot, and they deserve sympathy and support in this.

Even before this, however, First Aiders should take what steps they can to prevent secondary accidents by posting sentries, putting out warning signs and making themselves as conspicuously visible as they can.

The victims of road accidents may be thrown many yards and land out of sight, especially after dark. Similar scattering and concealment occurs on mountains, in mines and collapsing buildings, and with aircraft and railway accidents. A quick but careful search of the surroundings is important.

COMMON FATAL INJURIES

From 1 to 39 years of age more people die from accidents than from any one fatal disease (*Figure 2.1*), and the circumstances that most often carry the risk of fatal injuries are worth noting.

In persons of working age, head injuries and injuries of the trunk, often affecting several parts, are the main causes of death, which may be rapid. Table 2.1 shows that of the persons dying of such injuries in one large city, a third or more were dead on arrival in hospital.

In the lower part of the Table are the less frequent but rapidly fatal injuries and the frequent but less rapidly fatal consequences of injury.

TABLE 2.1
Causes of Death from Injury in One Large City in One Year

Main causes of death	Total number of deaths	Number of deaths before reaching hospital
Head injury	88	30
Multiple injuries	42	18
'Shock and haemorrhage'	25	11
Fracture of femur	42	7
Subsidiary causes of death		
Pulmonary embolism	17	2
Pneumonia following injury	79	1
Noxious gases	8	7
Miscellaneous causes	10	4

THE LETHAL EFFECTS OF INJURY

Bleeding and shock

Figure 2.2 shows the importance of bleeding after injuries of various parts of the body and the speed with which as much as half the 5 litres or so of blood in the average adult can be lost. These figures refer to injured people who survived long enough to reach hospital and have their blood volumes measured. Larger and more rapid losses occur in quickly fatal cases.

The speed and quantity of bleeding has an importance that varies with the age of the injured person. Weight for weight, children tolerate bleeding better than old people but because they have much smaller blood volumes will die rapidly from what may be negligible haemorrhage in the fully grown. For a given quantity of blood lost, the aged fare worse than young adults because their ability to compensate is less. *Figure 2.2* thus provides no more than evidence of what bleeding some adults can survive and it cannot be used to predict the outcome of any given haemorrhage. Nevertheless, it shows clearly the importance of haemorrhage. It has long been understood that haemorrhage is the most important cause of shock after injury, and it follows from this that First Aid is almost powerless in treating haemorrhagic shock, for which replenishment of the depleted circulation is necessary. It can, however,

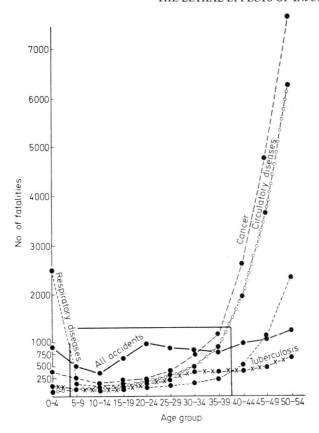

Figure 2.1. Accidents and other main causes of death

do much to limit and retard the progress of events caused by external bleeding. Usually nothing can be done to stop internal bleeding, but a suitable posture, avoiding disturbance, reducing pain and preventing chilling may help to mitigate its effects.

Injuries of the chest

First Aiders have a part in the treatment of shock caused by injuries of the chest. In some cases the cause is not bleeding but other influences on the action of the heart and respiratory organs. The circulation is

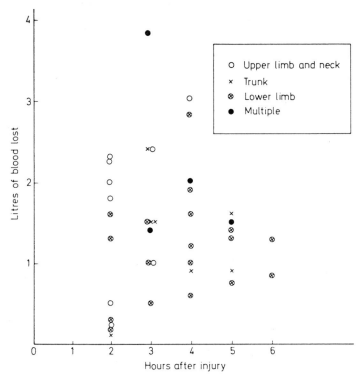

Figure 2.2. Speed and quantity of bleeding after various injuries

impaired but it may be a mechanical impairment, responsive to simple mechanical methods of treatment.

The current emphatic repetition of 'Treat for Shock' is admirable inasmuch as it keeps before the First Aider the fact that shock is serious and may develop insidiously or with dramatic suddenness, but it implies a much more effective role for First Aid in this respect than is suitable. 'Treat for Shock' is meaningful and proper advice to the doctor in hospital who has all that he needs, but it is misleading to the First Aider who may feel impelled to 'treat' the casualty instead of dispatching him without delay to those who can treat him.

Shock caused by burns and scalds is caused largely by a fall in the volume of blood in circulation and its treatment too is beyond First Aid. Shock caused by disease is outside the scope of this book.

Multiple injuries

With severe and multiple injuries the simple picture of haemorrhagic shock caused by a single serious injury is greatly complicated by the influences of the various injuries upon each other. Severe shock may mask serious injuries of the trunk; so may unconsciousness or a severed spinal cord. Profound haemorrhagic shock may cause unconsciousness because the reduced amount of haemoglobin available cannot supply the brain with the oxygen it needs (anaemic hypoxia). Severe injuries of the chest may do the same and for the same reason; they may also interfere with the oxygenation of a normal quantity of haemoglobin (hypoxic hypoxia) or with the free circulation of a normal quantity of fully oxygenated haemoglobin (stagnant hypoxia). There may be evident damage to the head but it is not necessarily responsible for an accompanying state of unconsciousness.

A good example of this sort of complex interaction was presented by the driver of a van in collision. She was at first conscious and 'not shocked' but soon became unconscious and on arrival in hospital about an hour later she had a systolic blood pressure of 40 mmHg, was profoundly unconscious, faintly cyanotic and breathing with slight stertor and paradoxical movement of the sternum and nearby chest wall. There was a faint bruise of the brow but no other sign of head injury. The profound shock suggested severe haemorrhage, possibly in the abdomen, and if so urgently requiring transfusion. On the other hand, the damage to the chest made it likely that injury of the lungs or heart was responsible for the shock and that transfusion would be dangerous. Was the unconsciousness caused by head injury, by hypoxia from oligaemia or by hypoxia from defective respiration? It transpired that bruising and a small puncture of the heart were most likely the key to the puzzle and the cause of both shock and unconsciousness.

Fortunately, the First Aider is not concerned with the niceties of clinical diagnosis in such a case. It is sufficient for him to recognize profound shock and loss of consciousness and to proceed accordingly, with the object of preserving life.

Suffocation

Impaired ventilation of the lungs is the other rapidly fatal consequence of injury and its importance has emerged with dramatic clarity in recent years. Much more can be done by First Aiders to treat this than to treat shock, and it is important to recognize the essential simplicity of the manner and causes of suffocation.

The object of breathing is to exchange gases between the atmosphere and the blood. Gases must therefore be both present and enabled to pass from alveoli to atmosphere. The refreshing movement of air in a building is referred to as ventilation, and it is helpful in clearing away the sense of awe and mystery induced in the lay mind by medical jargon to use a familiar term to denote a familiar process.

The air passages

Much emphasis has been laid, and rightly so, on artificial respiration, and no less detailed attention needs to be paid to ensuring a clear air passage before and during efforts to reproduce the movements of respiration. In spite of improved training it is still not an unusual experience to receive in hospitals persons whose limbs have been carefully splinted and whose wounds have been adequately dressed but whose breathing has been completely ignored.

Careful instruction in the physical signs of inadequate ventilation is obviously necessary but formal teaching is best driven home by practical experience. It is not easy to simulate defective ventilation in tests and competitions and though a First Aider may be well aware of its causes, signs and dangers when faced with an oral or written examination, he may not be presented with anything resembling it in competition work and may fail to recognize it in a genuine emergency.

It is an exaggeration to say that any person unconscious after injury has inadequate ventilation but it is a harmless one and, moreover, fully justified as an attempt to emphasize that the condition is frequent, often coming on insidiously and all too capable of ending fatally in a person whose brain could have recovered, given time and a good supply of fully oxygenated blood. It needs also to be clearly understood that when the visible parts of the body are affected by cyanosis, so is the brain and that a cyanotic brain is one in which any existing damage is being aggravated by the lack of oxygen of which cyanosis can be such a striking sign. It should also be mentioned that there can be a serious lack of oxygen in the body without even a trace of cyanosis and the lesson to be driven home is that clear and adequate breathing is the First Aider's most important objective in the unconscious casualty.

Drowning and gassing receive much attention in First Aid books but they are much less frequent than unconsciousness owing to head injury and injuries of the chest, which are therefore of much more practical importance as causes of inadequate ventilation.

A clear understanding of a few simple facts about inadequate ventilation is much more likely to save a life than is assiduously practised skill in applying artificial respiration.

The signs of suffocation

The physical signs of suffocation are fairly adequately set out in textbooks of First Aid but there is not enough guidance on the need to
suspect its occurrence and to look carefully for confirmation in its
early stages. Noisy breathing is obvious enough but cyanosis is not
easy for the unskilled to recognize in its early stages, especially in a
poor light or with dark or dirty skins. Frothing at the mouth is associated
by the layman with epileptic and other convulsions and with madness,
but it is not identified with the obstructed breathing that accompanies
these states. Recession of the intercostal spaces during inspiration is
an important sign that is easily recognized provided that it is sought. It
occurs at all ages but with the flexible chests of the young such marked
and extensive paradoxical movements can affect the sternum and the
costal cartilages so as to suggest widespread fractures.

There is no difficulty in teaching these signs but the important and
less easy task is to communicate the urgent need to look for them and
to recognize them and to presume some degree of suffocation in any
unconscious person.

Oxygen

This is rightly regarded as a valuable aid in dealing with hypoxia but
there is the danger that when available in an ambulance or First Aid
unit it will be used unnecessarily and incorrectly. In hospital it is by
no means unknown for oxygen to be administered because a patient is
cyanotic and without first ensuring that the cyanosis is not owing solely
to an obstructed air passage. If the air passages are clear, the 20 per cent
of oxygen in inspired air will usually prevent cyanosis: the success of
fresh air in this respect is too often ignored by those who have access
to oxygen.

Another frequent error is to direct oxygen towards the nose and
mouth by means of a tube and funnel instead of ensuring that the
patient breathes a high concentration of the gas through a suitable
and correctly applied mask or other device.

Carbon dioxide

In low concentration this gas stimulates the respiratory centre and has
been much used for this purpose, usually as a 5 per cent mixture in
oxygen. It is questionable whether carbon dioxide should ever be used

because when ventilation is defective the respiratory centre is already depressed by excessive carbon dioxide, or by hypoxia, or by both at once. In each case the patient needs adequate ventilation to expel the excess carbon dioxide and provide adequate oxygen. Coal gas poisoning requires a high concentration of oxygen to accelerate the expulsion of carbon monoxide from its association with haemoglobin. Carbon dioxide may be of value in such cases, but it is certainly dispensable.

ARTIFICIAL VENTILATION

The simplest and most effective method of artificial ventilation available for First Aid is direct inflation of the lungs by the expired air of a rescuer, which gives far better ventilation than the traditional methods of Schäfer, Silvester, Holger-Nielsen and others. Whereas, for example, Schäfer's method has provided a tidal volume of 250–600 ml, mouth-to-mouth ventilation can exchange a litre or more during each cycle.

The method of ventilation is fairly easy to apply even by the unskilled provided that the correct position of the patient is adopted. He must be supine with the neck well extended. The jaw can be held forwards by a thumb within the mouth but it is sufficient to support the chin by a hand below its point at the same time as the head is tilted fully but gently back. The rescuer's mouth is opened widely and applied round the mouth of the victim. If the victim is adult his nose is pinched; with a child the rescuer's mouth covers both nose and mouth of the victim. The chest can be seen to expand as the rescuer expires and to subside again as air is allowed to escape. Air is unlikely to enter the stomach if the neck is properly extended but should it do so, if an assistant is available he can apply pressure over the stomach to empty it and prevent further distension. There is, however, the risk that the patient will vomit and the rescuers should be prepared for this.

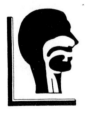 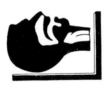 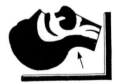

Head upright,   Head down,   After clearing pharynx of
partial obstruction   complete obstruction   mucus tilt head into
                                              sniffing position

Figure 2.3. A model in which movement of the neck alters the bore of the air passages
(From Dobkin, A.B. (1959). *Lancet* **2**, 662)

If for any reason it should be impossible to open the mouth, mouth-to-nose-ventilation can be carried out. In this case the jaw must be held forward by pressure applied behind its angle and the neck extended as before (*Figure 2.3*). Ventilation with expired air can be criticized on a number of grounds.

1. The supine position does not allow blood or other liquid to run out of the air passages. This is valid when there is continuing accumulation of liquid in the back of the nasopharynx because it may not be possible to clear this region properly by mopping out with a rag or swab.

2. It carries the risk of infection. The person at risk is the victim rather than his rescuer because the rescuer blows into the victim and withdraws as the victim exhales. This objection merits consideration but is not over-riding. The use of an inflatable model does not eliminate the risk of infection because the model can become a reservoir of exhaled germs of those using it. Makers' instructions for cleaning should be followed carefully.

3. The method is objectionable. This is true but when life is at stake the criticism loses much of its force. It is cogent, however, when training people in mouth-to-mouth ventilation but it is not necessary that training be carried further than describing the method and demonstrating the correct position of the patient, his neck and his jaw. Models can be used to provide experience of the effort necessary to inflate another person's lungs.

   Objections can be overcome by providing mouth-pieces that remove the rescuer's mouth from that of the victim, but such apparatus is not to be entrusted to the unskilled and possibly flustered First Aider. Another way of surmounting these objections is to use a small bellows and mask such as have been developed specially for this purpose. However, whatever its nature, unless apparatus is in working order and correctly used it may not only fail but be dangerous.

4. Expired air contains only 16 per cent oxygen as compared with the 20 per cent in the atmosphere. The difference is, in fact, not of practical importance because an active life can be led at 7,000 feet, where the head of pressure in oxygen is the same as in expired air. It is also worth noting that the cabins of high-flying aircraft have an atmospheric pressure equal to that at an altitude of about 8,000 feet.

5. Inflation of the lungs by pressure above that of the atmosphere in unphysiological: this is indeed so. The normal fall of pressure within the chest during inspiration assists the flow of venous

blood into the chest and so to the heart; during expiration the pressure-gradient is reversed and the return of blood consequently slowed. During mouth-to-mouth ventilation, the phase of the air-pressure curve is reversed and the minimum (slightly above atmospheric pressure) is at the end of expiration. The important consideration, however, is the difference between the inspiratory and expiratory pressures, which is certainly no less than with normal breathing. The mean pressure is a little higher, which means that the venous return will at first be reduced but as the new respiratory cycle becomes established venous flow will settle down to a more or less normal rate, though at slightly higher mean pressure than normal. Experience with intermittent positive pressure ventilation for long periods has established the value of the method. Inserting a sub-atmospheric phase widens the pressure-range and is beneficial in some conditions but this is irrelevant in First Aid.

6. Tilting the head back might be dangerous if the neck has been injured. This is a valid objection when there are signs of injury of the face and brow but extension of the neck should always be done gently; if there is any difficulty in doing it, the jaw should be held forward instead.

For the person whose face and neck are uninjured, mouth-to-mouth or mouth-to-nose ventilation is the most effective method available and it can be carried out whatever other injuries may be present and without assistance or apparatus. It is not tiring and can be continued for long periods even in awkward situations and positions. Care must be taken, however, not to ventilate excessively or the rescuer may become dizzy from overbreathing and the washing out from his own lungs of carbon dioxide.

If the jaws are broken or the face is badly wounded, it may be impossible to carry out this form of ventilation, even with a mouth-piece or mask. Apart from the difficulty of achieving an air-tight seal there may be profuse bleeding from the wounds of the mouth. The prone or semi-prone position should then be adopted because it allows the tongue and soft tissues to fall away from the pharynx and liquids in or entering it can run away.

In such circumstances one of the manual methods or the rocking method of Eve will have to be used. In spite of their relative ineffectuality they do ventilate the lungs and may suffice to tide the patient over until he breathes for himself or can be intubated.

Intubation provides a sure passage for artificial ventilation and may be performed from above through the nose or mouth or directly into the opened trachea. With a cuffed tube the lower air passages can be sealed off from blood, vomit or cerebrospinal fluid entering the pharynx. Gravity or suction help to drain the lower air passages. Tilting the patient's head downwards undoubtedly aids this process but it has been shown to cause the pressure within the skull to rise and so to reduce the flow of blood and oxygen to the brain. For the unconscious patient, therefore, any head-down tilt should be no more than sufficient to allow liquids to run out of the mouth instead of down the throat. If the coma or recovery position (*Figure 2.4*) is correctly used, tilting the head downwards should not be necessary.

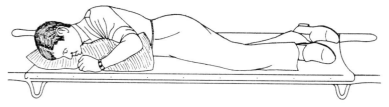

Figure 2.4. The coma position
(from Civil Defence Handbook No. 6, *First Aid* (1959) HMSO)

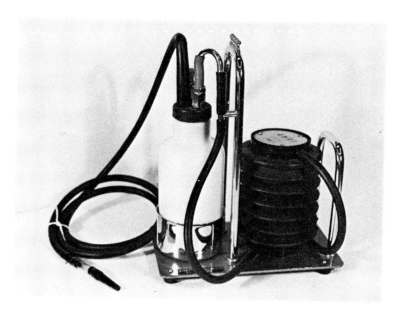

Figure 2.5. The Ambu pump

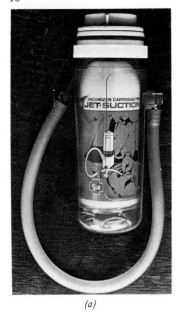

(a)

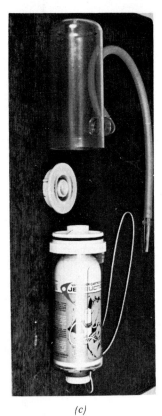

(c)

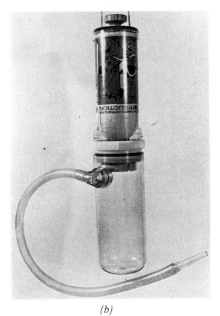

(b)

Figure 2.6. (a) The jet sucker packed up. (b) Assembled for use. Note the cord by which it can be hung from the neck. (c) The main component parts

Suction can be carried out successfully by means of the Ambu pump (*Figure 2.5*), but this is not easy to use on a soft or uneven surface or in a moving vehicle. A neat and effective device is the jet sucker (*Figure 2.6*), which hangs from the neck and provides 20 minutes of suction without loss of power.

Drowning

Drowning is perhaps the reason best known to the layman for applying artificial ventilation and although First Aid for the drowned has changed little over the years, our understanding of it has improved a good deal recently and some of the old ideas have been abandoned.

In the first place, a person does not have to inhale water in order to die as a result of immersion; dry drowning can occur, probably because of anoxia and reflex inhibition of the heart. In very cold water survival is measured in minutes (*Figure 2.7*) and death is caused

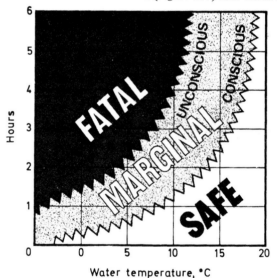

Figure 2.7. This graph showing approximate life expectancy in water in normal clothes was issued as part of a safety afloat drive
(from *Lifejackets and Personal Buoyancy Aids* 1973) by courtesy of RoSPA, 6 Buckingham Place, London, SW1)

by the intense chilling that occurs. Secondly, when water is inhaled it at once passes into the bloodstream. The lungs of drowned persons may be quite dry when examined at necropsy but if weed, silt or other irritant matter is inhaled it will cause intense irritation of the lungs and the outpouring of blood-tinged froth. Before inhaling water a drowned person swallows large quantities, which survivors have said relieves the urgent need to inhale. When water does run out of the mouth of a drowned person it comes from the stomach and not the lungs. The risk that this or other contents of the stomach may be regurgitated and inhaled must be borne in mind.

Another belief that has been shown to need revision is that the effects of drowning in fresh water differ in a number of ways from those of drowning in sea water, and particularly in being much more rapidly fatal. This belief arose from studying animals that had died of drowning. Those drowned in fresh water showed haemodilution and haemolysis, which killed the heart quickly by a combination of anoxia and the toxic effects of potassium from the burst cells. Drowning in sea water caused haemoconcentration but no haemolysis. More recent studies of human survivors have not shown these differences, which may be because the changes found after fatal incidents have not become fully established in those that have survived. What is important is that complete recovery has been known to follow over 20 minutes of complete immersion in fresh water. Such remarkable incidents may owe something to youthful victims and low temperatures but they reinforce the long-standing insistence that artificial ventilation should be started *as soon as the victim's head is above water* and without regard to the period of immersion. Even though such efforts may be less effective than those carried out on dry land or in a boat they may provide enough oxygen to maintain at least a spark of life until more forceful breaths can fan it into flame.

First Aid after drowning can be summarized as: artificial ventilation at the earliest possible moment; precautions against the effects of regurgitation from the stomach; and compressing the heart if no beat is detectable. Unlike ventilation of the lungs, this must wait until the victim can be laid on an unyielding surface. Finally, measures to overcome the effects of immersion and exposure must be taken (*see* page 253).

Because of the risks of pulmonary oedema, haemolysis and biochemical disturbance of the blood, persons rescued from drowning should be moved to hospital without delay and they should be given oxygen throughout the journey. If, as is likely, they are chilled they should be wrapped up but not warmed in any way. Such precautions are obviously necessary in cases of revival of those apparently dead from drowning but any persons known or thought to have inhaled even a small amount of water should be sent to hospital because they too can become victims of so-called secondary drowning. This can come on from a few minutes to several days after immersion and it is more likely to occur with salt-water than with fresh-water drowning.

Closely allied to drowning is the misfortune of being immersed while in a car. It has been taught that the wisest thing to do is to close all the windows and wait until water has ceased to enter, which will occur when the air trapped in the car has been compressed to the extent that it exerts as much pressure as that of the incumbent water. The doors can then be opened without difficulty. In the meantime those in the car have been able to breathe the trapped air and so can make their escape with fully aerated lungs. This theoretically plausible course of action has been found to be impracticable because trapped air is compressed to a much smaller volume than will allow respiration to continue. The wisest course is to leave the car with the least possible delay. Because the doors cannot be opened against the pressure of the water and because the weight of the engine will take most cars down nose first it has been suggested the easiest way to get out is by smashing the rear, or front, window (whichever is uppermost). The theoretical justification for this does not seem strong enough to overcome the practical difficulties of breaking a window under water and then trying to get through the jagged hole; getting out through an open side window seems more likely to be practicable, and to have the advantage of allowing up to four simultaneous escapes once the inrush of water has ceased.

Unless the vehicle falls into shallow water there is little prospect of successful rescue of any occupants from outside, but by the time a rescuer is able to reach the car and the doors can be opened, the occupants should be got out and brought to the surface as quickly as possible.

Gassing, electrocution and head injury

Artificial ventilation has an important part to play in resuscitating the victims of gassing, electrocution or head injury. In each case the heart may continue to beat after the respiratory centre has failed and, given enough oxygen, it can survive until the respiratory centre has become active again. If the rescuer cannot feel the apex beat of the heart or the carotid, aortic or femoral pulses he should assume that the heart has stopped beating and at once add attempts to restart it to the process of artificial ventilation.

RESTARTING THE HEART

A time-honoured stimulus to the heart is injecting adrenalin into it, but whether the efficient stimulus is mechanical or pharmacological is a matter of argument and for First Aid the question need not arise. A doctor may be present and may have needle and syringe with him but speed is all important as the brain is irrecoverably harmed by 3 to 4 minutes of anoxia.

1. Start artificial ventilation at once.
2. The patient should be supine and, if possible, on a hard surface.
3. Raise the legs to the vertical, unless injuries prevent this useful way of running blood back to the heart.
4. Strike the sternum sharply with the fist.
5. Press 60–70 times a minute with a fairly forcible jerky action applied to the lower part of the sternum, not the ribs. Having the patient on an unyielding surface makes it easier to squeeze the heart in this way.

The heart may begin to beat after any of these last three steps but its action may be feeble and fail and further efforts may be needed. It sometimes happens that a sharp blow on the sternum is followed by a regular heartbeat; it can also happen that the blow is followed by a single beat and that a second blow is followed by a second beat, and so on, even for half an hour or more. This is a very unusual state of affairs but when it does occur it has the great advantage that each heart beat is a natural one, albeit induced in an unnatural manner, with the result that a good circulation is maintained whereas when the heart is squeezed from without the circulation is much less than normal and special steps have to be taken to overcome increasing acidity of the blood. These are beyond the scope of First Aid. If there is no reaction to one or two sharp blows over the heart, external 'massage' should be started at once. This method of 'massage' has recently attracted a good deal of attention and has had a number of successes sometimes at the cost of broken ribs and injury of adjacent organs. Now that it has become part of standard First Aid its dangers must be stressed and the correct method must be clearly understood and taught.

Squeezing the heart through the open chest is scarcely to be regarded as First Aid, even for the doctor, especially now that externally applied pressure has been shown to be capable of maintaining some circulation even if the heart remains inert. The most important safeguard is to restrict pressure to the lower part of the sternum by pressing with the heel of one hand, the other hand being placed above it. Even in older persons the necessary 2.5–3.8 cm (1–1½ inches) depression of the sternum is quite easily achieved.

If single handed, the First Aider should start by clearing the air passage and inflating the lungs 5 or 6 times, then devote about 15 seconds to pressing the sternum and then alternate these actions until a second person is available.

It has to be admitted that the prospects of success appear from experience to be very small, but there is nothing to lose and even one life saved is a wonderful triumph. Success is most likely when a heart attack occurs in which the circulation to a fairly small part of the heart's muscle suddenly fails. If the heart does not stop beating altogether but begins the quivering action known as ventricular fibrillation the patient may die because effective circulation ceases. Squeezing the heart can keep the patient alive until other measures, such as electrical defibrillation, can be carried out and restore more normal action. A much more serious state of affairs exists when the heart stops all its activity and comes to a complete standstill known as asystole. Squeezing a heart in this condition is much less successful and electrical stimulation is without benefit. For the First Aider there is no way of distinguishing between asystole and fibrillation but 'cardiac

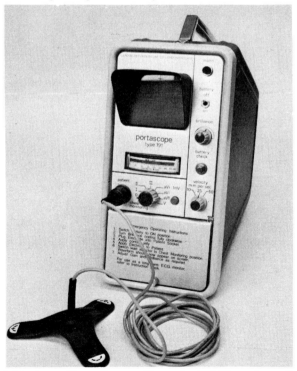

Figure 2.8 (a). A portable cardioscope. The tracing is visible on the small cathode ray tube at the top

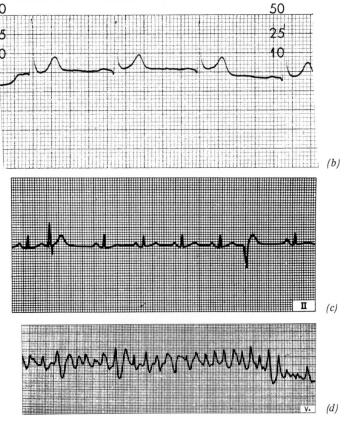

Figure 2.8 (b) Normal tracing. (c) Regular beats with abnormal pattern. (d) Ventricular fibrillation

flying-squads' carry apparatus for displaying the electrical action of the heart (*Figure 2.8*) and they can also carry out defibrillation and give drugs if necessary.

When the heart stops after serious injury, on the other hand, there is much less likelihood that it can be made to beat again because the cause of standstill is often exsanguination and no amount of massaging an empty heart will make it beat or set the blood successfully in motion again.

FIRST AID TO SAVE LIFE

1. External haemorrhage must be stopped (*see* Chapter 4).
2. Obstruction to breathing must be overcome. Clearing the pharynx

by hand and placing the patient prone or semi-prone with the mouth and nose free will usually suffice for the unconscious patient who is still breathing.

3. Artificial ventilation should then be started at once if breathing has ceased. Mouth-to-mouth or mouth-to-nose ventilation gives the best exchange of gases. It may be dangerous if the neck is thought to have been broken and unsatisfactory if there is much liquid (blood, cerebrospinal fluid or vomitus) accumulating in the pharynx. It may be difficult or impossible to carry out effectively if the face or jaws have been badly injured.

For the doctor there is a place for intubation, even tracheostomy. Tracheostomy is used to ensure a clear air passage by short-circuiting obstruction and by allowing the air passages to be emptied by suction. In an emergency it should be used for the former purpose only, for example, with laryngeal oedema or spasm and with impacted food or other matter. Apparatus intended to facilitate tracheostomy or laryngotomy is unlikely to be either safe or successful except in experienced hands. Intubation of the trachea by way of the nose or, preferably, the mouth requires a good deal of skill and practice as well as suitable apparatus (*Figure 2.9*). It can be carried out only on a person who is

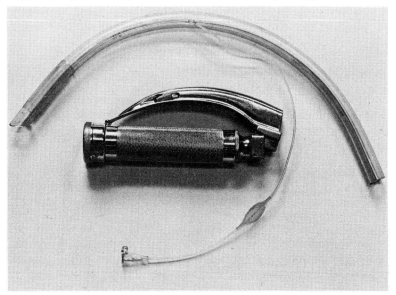

Figure 2.9. Endotracheal tube and a laryngoscope

deeply unconscious or completely relaxed by anaesthesia and the greatest difficulties arise when it is most urgently needed. It was found to be possible to take completely unskilled persons and teach them how to intubate the human trachea but it was also found that few could maintain their ability to do so without frequent practice and there were those that were successful in the classroom but lacked the confidence to make an attempt when it was urgently necessary for them to do so.

Other causes of defective ventilation will be dealt with in the section dealing with injuries of the chest (*see* Chapter 9).

LETHAL CAUSES OF INJURY

The First Aider must remove lethal causes of injury from the patient or remove the patient from them.

The main dangers come from poisonous fumes and gases, electric currents, burning and crushing, either existing or imminent. The hazards of a noxious atmosphere and electric currents need little comment as they are well recognized in books on First Aid, but there is the possibility of carrying out artificial ventilation in a noxious atmosphere. This subject began to receive attention when 'nerve gases' were introduced. These agents are anticholinesterases and are destroyed fairly quickly in the body provided that the victim can be kept alive. The need is for a supply of uncontaminated air. This can be provided by a rescuer wearing a gas-mask but he must be able to expire to the victim. It is not enough to apply a mask to the victim and to connect the two, because the pressure required to fill the victim's lungs is higher than the escape pressure between the face and the mask. An attempt has been made to overcome this difficulty by providing the rescuer with a special expiratory tube and mouth-piece. He breathes in through his mask in the usual way but breathes out through the expiratory tube, which leads to the victim, who does not need a mask. Equipment of this sort is not generally available and all that can be done at present is to remove a gassed person from a noxious atmosphere and to carry out artificial ventilation as soon as possible. It may be tempting to apply a spare mask, if available, to a casualty and then to carry out artificial ventilation, but the dead space in the air passages and mask is about the same as the tidal volume that manual methods of ventilation can achieve. An available mask should, of course, be applied if the gassed person is still breathing and kept on until fresh air is available.

The trapped casualty

A person who has been trapped by wreckage of any kind poses a number of problems. The most important decision is whether his life is immediately endangered. This applies to burning and the risk of explosion, to crushing of the head, chest or abdomen or the likelihood that this will occur at any moment, and to inadequately accessible victims of severe bleeding and suffocation. In these conditions speedy and more or less forcible extraction is justified even though it may carry the risk of aggravating existing injuries or inflicting fresh ones. Because of these risks, however, frantic haste is undesirable when the victim is not in immediate danger of his life.

The crush syndrome

This results from severe and prolonged crushing of limbs. It is characterized by renal failure consequent upon the profound hypotension that is caused by great loss of circulating blood into the crushed tissues after they have been released. The previous emphasis on the part played by myoglobin and other products of disrupted tissues was misplaced. These products can be present without detriment to the kidney provided that the blood pressure is restored quickly to normal by liberal transfusion of blood. The longer a limb has been crushed the greater the likelihood that the crush syndrome will develop, but there is not the same urgency to extricate the victim as with, for example, a severely crushed chest. If the limb has been crushed for 3 or 4 hours or more or is so badly injured as to be irrecoverable, a very tight tourniquet should be applied as near as possible to the proximal edge of the crushed part, preferably before release. This tourniquet can be left in place until the limb is amputated, which may be necessary to free the patient. This policy prevents the loss of liquids into the crushed part and the escape into the bloodstream of myoglobin and other products of anoxia and injury. If the limb has been crushed for a short time and is thought to be capable of recovery and of being repaired, it should be firmly bandaged—other injuries permitting—so as to try and prevent excessive swelling. A tourniquet should not be used unless there is severe bleeding that cannot be controlled in any other way.

It is recommended that victims of crushing be made to drink copiously. This should be ignored if the crushed part has been amputated or excluded by a tight tourniquet or if the victim will reach hospital within 10 to 15 minutes or so. If there will be much delay, drinking may be allowed. Small quantities should be given at first and larger quantities only if there is no vomiting. The liquid absorbed is freely diffusible through the walls of capillaries and will do virtually nothing to raise the blood pressure, though it will help to replenish the body's depleted stock of water. Plain or flavoured water, tea or other beverages are equally permissible; none has any great advantage over others.

First Aiders are liable to over-dramatize and one has known of a person with a squashed hand being urged to drink several pints of water. The crush syndrome only occurs after severe and prolonged crushing of large masses of muscle in the limbs.

Extrication

There is little recorded information on how this is carried out or about its effects. Although rescue squads must be well aware of the difficulties,

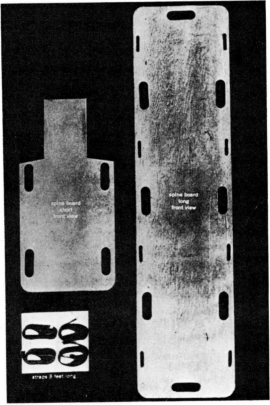

Figure 2.10. Dr Farrington's spinal boards, which are firmly held to the patient by stout straps passed through the slots

they do not necessarily recognize the dangers accompanying the often unceremonious hauling of injured people from wreckage and danger or realize when delay is desirable to enable the trapped person to be freed more gently. The pioneering efforts of Dr Farrington in the United States of America include the introduction of a spinal board for the safe removal of casualties from vehicles (*Figure 2.10*). The casualty is firmly secured by stout webbing straps that pass round the top of each thigh, cross in front of the body and are firmly anchored in the slots. The neck is supported by a ready-made collar or one improvised from a folded-up newspaper and the head is bound firmly to the narrow part of the board. An important characteristic of such a board is a smooth surface that will make it possible to slide it between the casualty and the back of the seat. Properly applied, this board provides protection for all parts of the spine. Nevertheless, First Aiders should be urged to note the general condition of the victim before and after extraction and to report any observation that leads them to believe that injuries have been aggravated or inflicted in the process.

FACILITATING DEFINITIVE TREATMENT

Apart from saving life much can be done to help, or hinder, successful care in hospital.

In the beginnings of First Aid there was often not much difference between the treatment that could be provided at the scene of injury and that available in hospital. Doctors relied heavily on natural powers of healing. It was accepted that wounds would inevitably suppurate and hoped that the pus would be thick and creamy—laudable because the staphylococci usually responsible were less likely to kill the patient than the more invasive streptococci or clostridia that resulted in thin or sanious discharge. The definitive treatment of a wound was simply a matter of dressing and awaiting healing, aided if necessary by drainage of deep collections of pus and the removal of sequestra. The only other surgical measures were the use of ligatures and amputation.

With the present emphasis on preventing infection, First Aid must be content with providing proper cover and avoiding other methods of local treatment. The individual is often unable to provide adequate dressing but he can at least refrain from messing up the wound. This subject is dealt with in detail in the next chapter.

In the case of fractures, a much more active policy of treatment has been adopted and direct surgical attack upon the broken bones is not unusual. Most fractures will unite if left entirely alone and human remains from bygone ages have confirmed this, though malunion was the rule.

Former methods of splintage did little but steady the limb; accurate replacement and effectual immobilization of the fragments were often impossible with the crude appliances previously available. The surgeon relied upon the clinically determinable strength of union and the patient's preparedness to use the limb to decide the length of treatment. Against this background the use by the First Aider of ready-made or improvised splints enabled him to do almost as much for the fracture initially as was within the power of the experienced surgeon.

Nowadays, the First Aider's efforts compare less favourably because fractures can be so much better treated by doctors. He should be content to render the limb comfortable and to steady it enough to allow a casualty to be transported without undue disturbance and pain. This is all that is required to stay the progress of shock from these injuries; formal splintage is not necessarily the best way of achieving these objectives but inflatable splints offer a valuable combination of simplicity, comfort and efficacy. Any wound must be covered.

The First Aider may have to dress wounds. He must also be clearly aware of the dangers of fractures, know how to recognize the dangers and how to mitigate them. He should prevent a closed fracture from becoming open; recognize when the circulation to a limb has been imperilled and have some safe idea of how to set about improving it; recognize the likelihood that important organs and structures may have been injured or may be in danger and know how to reduce that danger.

To the First Aider, this emphasis on 'don't' is in unwelcome contrast to the elaborate methods of splintage that have been laid down in the past. The recent recognition in the First Aid manuals that formal splintage is not the be-all and end-all of fracture treatment is overdue but could be carried further with advantage. It is not unusual for First Aid workers to point a gently accusing finger at the medical profession because a doctor at the scene of an accident is not always the most active attendant to the patient's injuries. Whilst it is true that many doctors have only a sketchy knowledge of First Aid teaching that does not mean that they are useless in an emergency or incapable of improvising unorthodox but useful treatment. Indeed in many parts of the country doctors have trained and equipped themselves to provide a very high standard of First Aid, even before the ambulance arrives in some cases. Useful treatment is one thing but a determined attempt to fill in (sometimes waste) time by lavishing 'treatment' on any and every injury is not always preferable to well-judged restraint or even masterly inactivity.

The reasons for splinting fractures and the way in which broken limbs should be handled and secured is dealt with in Chapter 5.

SUMMARY

First Aid can do much to preserve life in an emergency and strenuously active measures may be required. When it comes to facilitating definitive treatment a more passive role will often serve the patient best. When to act and when to stand by can best be decided if the benefits of activity and observation are soundly based on an understanding of the nature of the injuries and their dangers and of the beneficial part that First Aid has to play. The First Aider has a particularly valuable contribution to make when he pays discerning attention to the circumstances and consequences of the accident and can render a report to those to whom he surrenders his responsibility.

3

WOUNDS

A wound is a break in the continuity of tissues and is fundamentally a destructive injury. It frequently includes a breach of the surface layer of skin or mucous membrane and thus becomes exposed to the risk of infection, which may disastrously complicate an already severe wound or gravely dominate a trivial one. The management of wounds thus centres upon repair of the damage and prevention or treatment of infection.

INFECTION

Terminology

Various terms are used to describe the presence and effects of bacteria in wounds and require definition.

Contamination

The demonstrable presence of bacteria in a wound without any of the signs of active inflammation, such as heat, redness, swelling, pain, loss of function and suppuration. This term is usually restricted to the presence of bacteria in wounds that are but a few hours old. When bacteria are found in older but apparently healthy wounds, then the term colonization has been used.

Infection

Bacteria are present and the wound is inflamed.

These terms are based on a bacteriologist's report on cultures made from the wounds; it is also convenient to have descriptions of the appearance of wounds.

Sepsis

Inflammation, suppuration and perhaps sloughs are present, irrespective of bacteria. Septic, that is, messy-looking wounds are not invariably populated by pathogenic organisms. Clean-looking wounds, on the other hand, may yield them in profusion.

General considerations

In most instances infection enters through the breached surface layer but it can also arrive by way of the bloodstream and, rarely, by bacterial permeation of an injured but unbroken surface. Even when the skin has been penetrated this may have occurred without being recognized at the time: it has been found that about a third of the septic hands and fingers treated in industrial firms' accident rooms occurred without known injury. It follows from this that not all infections can be prevented; an outstanding example is tetanus, which rarely follows large wounds and may occur in the absence of any known break in the skin. Nevertheless, much can be done to prevent infection if there is a clearer understanding of the process than most First Aiders possess.

The skin has the ability to cleanse itself and this ability lies partly in its fatty secretions but the process of self-cleaning is so slow that it is always lagging behind the continual process of contamination by bacteria and cannot be put to practical use.

The bacterial population includes both pathogenic and harmless organisms and is influenced by the environment, occupation and habits of the individual. Of the pathogenic organisms, *Staphylococcus aureus* is the most important. It inhabits the noses of about 30 per cent of normal, healthy people and the perinea of about 10 per cent. From these sources it spreads, or is conveyed, to the skin, hair, hands, clothing, and farther afield through the air, mainly by way of dust. *Clostridium welchii* often occurs on the skin but causes infection only with exceptional rarity in civilian life. This is largely because relatively few injuries damage muscle seriously, because gas gangrene is usually the result of infection by several different clostridia in company and because wounds are usually treated both promptly and adequately. Streptococci are occasionally found in the throats of healthy people, but only rarely on healthy skin.

Generally speaking, dry skin is more resistant to infection than moist skin and friction adds to the likelihood of infection.

Self-infection

It follows from this that as soon as a wound is inflicted it may be contaminated by the patient's own bacterial population. In most cases only a few of these bacteria enter a wound during the first hour or two and even pathogenic organisms do not establish themselves in less than a few hours.

Apart from the patient's own skin and other reservoirs of organisms, bacteria may come from his clothing and other materials, some of which may be driven deeply into the tissues. This is a particularly dangerous state of affairs because this sort of foreign material is likely to be densely populated by the patient's own bacteria and by others derived from elsewhere.

Added infection

Foreign matter varies greatly in its capacity to cause infection. Metal fragments from a machining process, for example, are often nearly sterile whereas soil, road dirt and vegetable matter are usually heavily contaminated. Small arms' bullets are not, as has been supposed, automatically sterilized by their speed of flight. Direct implantation of bacteria is also the result of careless handling of sterile instruments and dressings, or the use of unsterile materials, especially in primitive communities where dung is regarded as a sovereign remedy and the consequent high mortality and morbidity rates are accepted as part of the established order of things. Civilized man may pride himself on his superior knowledge of these matters but there is not all that much justification for pride when one considers the amount of infection against the background of knowledge and facilities that are available.

Medicaments

The pressure exerted by advertisements on the lay, and also on the medical, man maintains the age-old belief in the value of substances applied to wounds and other injuries. We have passed from the era of salves and balms to the era of disinfectants and antiseptics; we are now in the era of 'scientific' preparations such as antibiotics and hormones. The effectiveness of these agents to prevent and treat infection has increased with each stage but they have a common danger in that they are applied to the injured surface. Correctly done this can be advantageous and achieve the desired effect but it is too little understood that infection or secondary infection is likely to follow sooner or later. It has been found, for example, that unskilled attempts to cleanse or 'sterilize' a wound can result in a richer growth of organisms than the mere application of a sterile, or even a clean, dry dressing.

Antiseptics and disinfectants kill organisms by denaturing the proteins in their protoplasm. It is not always appreciated by the medical man and is entirely beyond the knowledge of most laymen that what harms the protoplasm of bacteria is not the most innocuous substance to apply to the protoplasm of the cells exposed in the wound—cells that have the capacity to kill and ingest bacteria and to carry out the process of healing, provided that they are not harmed. The use of sulphonamides and antibiotics on wounds has become widespread, but because it carries the risk of adding bacteria to a wound it is to be condemned unless carried out with the facilities for accurate bacteriological control that exist only in hospitals.

The First Aider must content himself with applying nothing more than a clean or, if available, a sterile covering to the wound. All medicaments should be forbidden. As soon as a wound is inflicted the risk of infection exists and this risk will continue until the wound has been securely closed. It can be reduced but not abolished by the intelligent use of coverings or dressings. There are various made-up and sterile dressings (*Figure 3.1*). Failing these, a clean cloth, preferably recently laundered, will do. The traditional handkerchief or torn-up shirt may be

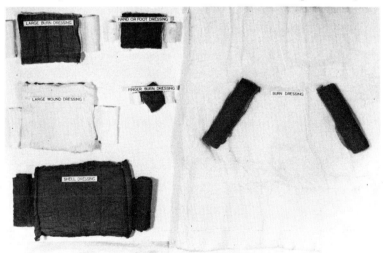

Figure 3.1. Standard dressings of First Aid kits

a self-sacrificing offering but is likely to carry with it a goodly crop of the donor's bacterial flora. For really large wounds (*Figure 3.2*) it is usually necessary to improvise. With the co-operation of hospitals and other bodies it may be possible to make dressings 46 cm (18 inches) or so square by stitching a double thickness of Gamgee tissue on to sterilizable and waterproof paper (*Figure 3.3*). The fringe of paper is

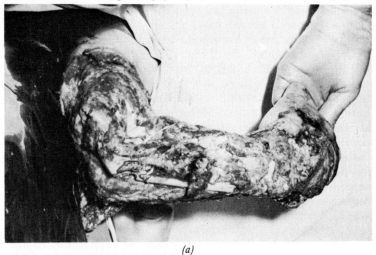

(a)

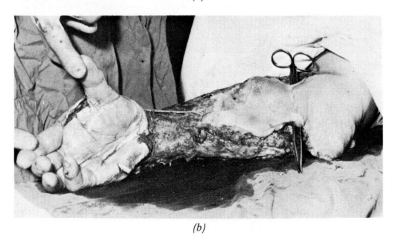

(b)

Figure 3.2 (a) (b). Very severe injury including extensive loss of skin caused when the limb was dragged along under an overturned motor car. There was still useful function in the hand and the limb could be saved

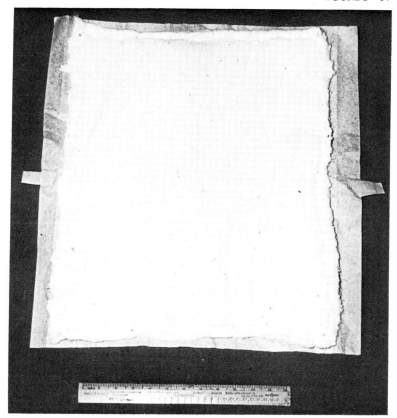

Figure 3.3. A home-made dressing 41 cm (16 inches) square. A double layer of Gamgee tissue is stitched to sterilizable, waterproof paper, which is on the outside when the dressing is folded for packing

useful for handling the dressing, which can be kept in place by triangular bandages, an inflatable splint or other means. Stitching on tapes for this purpose does not make the dressing any easier to handle or secure.

Other influences promoting infection

Healthy tissues have considerable power to overcome contaminant bacteria and to halt infection. This they achieve by virtue of the lytic and phagocytic properties of the cells scattered throughout the tissues and conveyed by the blood. The cells are aided by the specific antibodies produced by the reticulo-endothelial system. In each case, however, the antibacterial effectiveness of these second and third lines of defence (the skin being the first) depends upon the defences' having direct access to the invaders. Anything that intervenes favours the invaders. Dead and devitalized tissue (which includes blood shed into the spaces of the wound) provides contaminant bacteria with an excellent culture medium and with a refuge from the cellular and humoral defenders.

Tissues injured by the wounding agent may die at once or they may survive for hours or days until overcome by arrest of the local circulation. All injuries cause some local swelling and though often mild and transient it may be sufficient to compress the small vessels and slow the circulation. Resulting hypoxia increases the permeability of the capillaries, exudation occurs and swelling increases. The circulation is further hampered and may ultimately cease. The stage is set for bacterial contamination to develop into infection, which may in turn increase the area of gangrene by swelling and septic thrombosis.

Injuries that divide tissues without otherwise harming them have been described as tidy and usually heal well if properly treated. Injuries in which tissues have been crushed, tattered and torn have been described as untidy and are much more likely to heal poorly and to become infected.

HEALING

Healing starts as an inflammatory response to injury and is later characterized by the transformation of cells from the reticulo-endothelial system into new blood vessels and fibroblasts, which seal the breach. It follows that the smaller the breach is, or can be made, the more quickly will it be sealed. Rapid healing is best shown in the incised surgical wound. This is a tidy wound in which the tissues are cleanly divided and then brought closely together by stitches and held there until securely united by scar. A sharp knife inflicts little damage other than the division of tissues.

It is the aim of surgery to make all wounds as nearly tidy as possible by removing dead and damaged tissue and bringing the remaining viable tissues snugly together. The breach is thereby reduced to a narrow cleft that will quickly be spanned by the fibroblastic reaction in its walls, unhampered by inert matter and able to deal with all but heavy bacterial contamination.

This aim is not always attainable because the viability of tissues cannot always be determined at the time of operation. The effects of swelling and thrombosis take time to declare themselves and any estimate of viability is necessarily tentative within the first few hours after injury. It is a matter of common experience that an accidental, incised wound that has been properly treated usually heals promptly without swelling, pinkness or exudation, whereas a wound that has been lacerated or contused shows these signs of impeded healing.

THE PRACTICAL APPLICATIONS OF THE PRINCIPLES OF TREATMENT

FRESH WOUNDS

Immediate steps

Severe bleeding must be stopped (*see* Chapter 4). Obvious foreign matter must be removed if possible. It may be permissible to take hold of clothing or a projecting piece of wood or glass with the fingers and try to remove it, but only if the fingers will not touch the wound. Grit and gravel can be removed by wiping with a sterile dressing or picked out with sterile forceps, if either is available. Otherwise, it is better to leave foreign matter alone and to apply a dressing over it if the patient will reach skilled care soon.

Air embolism is a rare complication of some wounds, particularly those in the neck, where if a large vein has been pierced air may be drawn into it during inspiration. The result is that the heart contracts ineffectually on bloody froth, and death soon follows. Any wound that is noticed to have air passing inwards or outwards must be dressed without delay and if the patient is in dire straits the wound should be plugged immediately with whatever is available and sufficient for the purpose—handkerchief, glove, even the bare fist. Air is less likely to enter veins if the injured part is kept below the level of the heart, even though this may make it more difficult to staunch bleeding from the neck, for example.

Attempts to cleanse the injured part or to 'sterilize' the wound by applying medicaments are generally undesirable. There is, however, no harm in putting a small cut under the tap because tap water is reasonably free from pathogenic bacteria and the ensuing bleeding helps to irrigate the wound from within.

In primitive countries or if skilled care will necessarily be delayed for many hours, careful wiping of the skin around the wound with cloths that have been boiled and allowed to cool helps to remove dirt, blood and contaminating bacteria. Once the skin has been cleansed, with a fresh piece of cloth for each wipe, other fresh pieces can be used gently on the wound itself and some of the boiled, but suitably cool water poured over it. The pieces of cloth should be handled with instruments that have been boiled or flamed.

Water is harmless: the same cannot always be said of the many preparations that have been advocated and used for the purpose of cleansing a wound.

Limbs that are caught between rollers or run over by rubber tyres are liable to suffer very severe injuries in which the skin is widely split and stripped from the tissues beneath (*Figure 3.4*). Large flaps may be kinked and twisted. They should be gently laid back in place so as to relieve the obstruction of their circulation that distortion can cause. Much of the skin may die but what survives is sometimes of great value and the amount that does survive is sometimes much greater than could have been expected. Whether or not the area is cleansed or merely dressed will depend upon the speed with which skilled care can be provided. Unless careful surgical treatment can be carried out within a few hours, the stripped skin is likely to die entirely and the survival of the limb itself may be doubtful.

Rollers and tyres can inflict comparably severe injuries without breaking the skin; nevertheless the skin has been damaged and as it becomes distended by the bleeding within it may begin to blister. Decompression is indicated but the most that the First Aider can do is to apply a firm supporting bandage over the whole injured part and get the patient to hospital as soon as possible.

Sometimes there are severely damaged pieces of tissue that are almost free or are obviously beyond hope of recovery. In a hot, dry climate exposed tissues dry rapidly and loose masses of skin, muscle or tendon that have become hard, brown and dry can be cut away with sterilized knife, razor-blade or scissors. They need not be saved, except to show what has been done. This course of action is appropriate and desirable in some circumstances, but clearly if it is to be recommended to the First Aider in a primitive community great caution must be observed by the teacher and enjoined upon the First Aider.

Separate parts can sometimes be utilized and should therefore be preserved, preferably in clean or sterile dressings. A completely avulsed scalp is of little use because it requires more nourishment than it can obtain when replaced as a free graft. If any exposed surface is allowed to dry it will die and not support a graft, but it is not necessary to apply moist dressings for the discharge from the wound will keep it moist if it is covered.

Large pieces of bone have proved useful; after being boiled and replaced they can provide a useful natural scaffolding that may prevent what would otherwise be severe deformity. Much larger parts, even

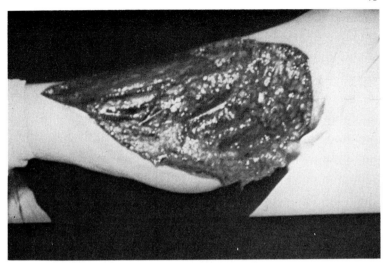

Figure 3.4 (a). A flap of skin torn loose and crumpled (cont.)

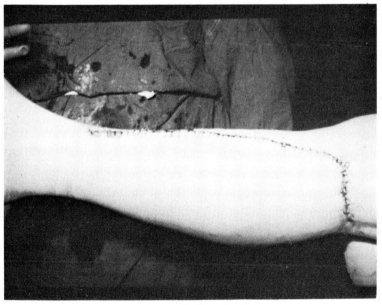

Figure 3.4 (b). Some of it died after being sewn back

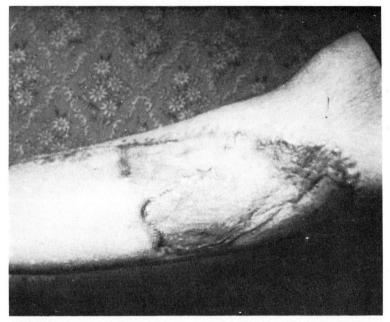

Figure 3.4 (c). The dead skin was cut away and Thiersch grafts laid in its place

entire limbs, should also be sent to hospital because it may be worth re-attaching them. Where there is any prospect of success this is increased by keeping the severed part as cold as possible, with ice-water if possible, and making both it and the patient available for operation at the earliest possible moment. Ice-water may contain large numbers of bacteria but it may be possible to seal the severed part in a plastic bag and then immerse it. The technique of re-attachment has been worked out and a number of useful extremities have been restored. Although the opportunities for replacing separated parts and tissues are few they cannot exist at all unless First Aiders provide them for consideration. If there is any possibility of re-attaching part of the body it may be helpful for the hospital to be given prior notice so that the elaborate preparations can be started if necessary and in good time.

Dressing

Dry gauze, Gamgee tissue or smooth fabric may be applied to the wounds, but never wool. For many of the wounds that the First Aider is called upon to treat the small prepared dressings that include adhesive plaster are adequate, but for the larger wounds improvisation is necessary.

Outside the gauze there should be a layer of absorbent material sufficiently thick to take up the wound's exudate without becoming soaked through. This should be kept firmly in place by bandaging. The ideal bandage is crape, which can be made to exert firm, even pressure and will do much to stop bleeding. Cotton, triangular and improvised bandages cannot be expected to do much more than keep the dressing in place and, especially in the hands of the unskilled, they are not suitable for applying firm pressure. It should be mentioned that the larger the bulk of dressing material the more blood it can absorb. A piece of Gamgee tissue 41 cm (16 inches) square will hold roughly two donations of blood without dripping. If, therefore, such a dressing is seen to have blood soaking through to the surface it is a warning that noteworthy bleeding is still going on.

The main object of the dressing is to prevent contamination of the wound by exposure to the air and by contact with clothing and the like. It will fail in this object if it is not itself sterile and if it slips. It may fail if it becomes soaked through because bacteria can grow inwards or outwards through soaked dressings, but provided that the dressing is thick and can soon be changed, bacteria from without will not penetrate to the wound.

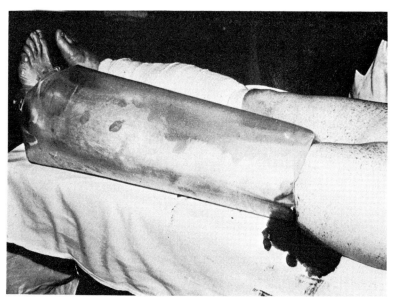

Figure 3.5. Steady bleeding continued from an open fracture that was comfortably supported by an inflatable splint

The subject of wounds and dressings should not be set aside without considering the benefit of applying some of the available dressings, which may be too small to cover the wound or are so ill placed or ill secured that they do not in any sense cover or protect the wound. In general, it is only realistic to suggest that if it is not possible to cover a wound completely with the dressings available there is little point in merely going through the motions of applying a dressing, with one exception. That is when there is need to apply pressure to a bleeding point.

Another means of covering a wound of an extremity is to enclose the part in a sterile, impermeable bag. This eliminates the problems of soaking and of providing large quantities of sterile wool, for packing is applied outside the bag. Any soft material can be used, such as clothing, mechanic's waste or grass, with a bandage applied over all. This method has not been used much but has the obvious advantage that the essential feature—the bag—is readily available commercially in different sizes and takes up little space. The other dressing materials can be improvised. The inflatable splint can be used in much the same way but it is not sterile and it does not stop bleeding (*Figure 3.5*).

Drugs

Except in hospital, where proper precautions can be taken and bacteriological control provided, nothing but a dry dressing should be applied to a wound. The First Aid worker will not ordinarily have access to antibacterial drugs that can be given by mouth or by injection but in primitive communities these may be available to the semi-skilled and even the unskilled and their use, and abuse, deserves consideration.

If the patient will receive skilled care within a few hours of injury, it is doubtful whether there is any great advantage in enhanced antibacterial powers. Antitoxin still has a place in under-doctored areas because poor hygiene increases the risk of tetanus and infrequent recourse to doctors makes repeated doses unlikely. Nevertheless, if anti-tetanus serum is given, due precautions must be taken against precipitating anaphylaxis. If the patient has had a previous injection of serum, 0.2 ml should be given subcutaneously. If there has been no general disturbance in 20—30 minutes the rest of the dose should be given intramuscularly. If there is a history of allergy the serum should be diluted by 9 volumes of saline solution and 0.2 ml of the dilute serum given subcutaneously. If there has been no general reaction 20—30 minutes later, 0.2 ml of undiluted serum should be injected into the subcutaneous fat and a further period of 20—30 minutes allowed to elapse without disturbance before giving the full dose.

The preliminary injections are test doses in the sense that they test the person's general sensitivity. Local redness and swelling are no guide to general sensitivity and may be ignored. The purpose of the test doses is to enable the effect of a small dose, slowly absorbed, to be studied. Should anaphylaxis ensue it may have a sufficiently gradual onset to allow treatment to be carried out in time to avoid a fatal reaction. The safest antitoxin is prepared with human serum but it is scarce and expensive.

There is little place for antitoxin in the prevention of tetanus in well-doctored areas, where it is now known that the dangers and shortcomings of repeated doses of anti-tetanic serum make it second best to active immunity induced by tetanus toxoid: to confer immunity this has to be given in 3 doses at respective intervals of 6–12 weeks and 6–12 months. Immunity is maintained by further doses at intervals of 5–10 years or after further injury. Except in those already actively immune a single dose offers no protection. Whenever possible the state of immunity should be ascertained and whenever appropriate toxoid should be given to a wounded person. For this purpose a national campaign of active immunization and a nationally recognized token of active immunity induced by tetanus toxoid: to confer immunity this person's immunity to tetanus, penicillin, erthyromycin or tetracyclines are used in an attempt to offer immediate protection.

Anti-gas gangrene serum is of doubtful value and is much less used than formerly. It too carries the risk of anaphlyaxis.

Referring the patient to a doctor

The surface appearance of a wound is an unreliable guide to its importance. Even scratches, grazes and pricks have been followed by severe and sometimes fatal septicaemia or tetanus. It is unrealistic to insist that all such apparent trivialities be sent to a doctor and it is by no means certain that skilled medical attention would, in fact, prevent occasional disasters. Washing under a tap, a dry dressing and instructions to report at once should there by any swelling, redness or throbbing is adequate treatment in the first instance. Signs of infection demand medical advice.

The most important decisions concern small and innocent-looking cuts and punctures. These should receive the attention of a doctor, especially when they affect the scalp, hands, trunk or the neighbourhood of joints and great vessels. The history may be of decisive importance. Wounds inflicted by deliberate or accidental stabbing, or in the course of a fall or road accident have had considerable force behind them and should be presumed in the first place to have penetrated dangerously.

Scalp wounds may be trivial in appearance but overlie a depressed fracture, for which surgical exploration is required. Hair may be trapped in the fracture-line and the dura mater may be torn.

Unexpectedly large objects can pass through disconcertingly small wounds. A car's door handle penetrated the skull of a child and was recognized only because the child was unconscious and was radiographed. The handle was removed successfully after the small wound had been greatly enlarged. A soldier thought he had suffered a glancing blow from a bullet; there was a small wound in front of the ear and a 20 mm shell in the nasopharynx. A cyclist fell off his machine and inflicted a small wound on his knee. Several inches of the blade of a screwdriver had embedded itself in the lower end of the femur and snapped off.

Cuts on the hand and fingers do not have to be very deep to injure nerves or tendons or to open joints. The First Aider may notice deformity or loss of movement or feelings and these are clear signs that something more than a dressing is needed. It must be stressed, however, that apparently normal function does not rule out serious damage. A finger can be moved even though a tendon has been largely divided or a joint opened. Synovial liquid is occasionally seen to exude from a wound that has entered a joint or tendon sheath.

Stab wounds are an occupational hazard among butchers, wood workers and leather workers who use sharp knives. The alleged depth of a penetration is usually a gross underestimate, and a 'nick' in the groin or abdominal wall has too often inflicted grave injury on main blood vessels of the bowel to be left unexplored. There may at first be no sign whatever that a mortal wound has been sustained. People have been known to walk several hundred yards after a stab-wound of the heart, to be sent away with a sticking plaster on the abdomen to die of peritonitis from a perforated bowel, or with a dressing on the groin to develop an arteriovenous fistula.

Cut throat is an alarming condition that can lay bare many important structures in the neck without harming any. Such wounds should be dressed in the usual way and the patient given no chance to make a more thorough attempt at suicide. When there is profuse bleeding life is in danger from this and perhaps from air embolism. A natural reaction is to apply a firm dressing to the bleeding place. However, such a wound may have divided the trachea, which means that a dressing sometimes has to be applied so that it will stop bleeding without blocking the air passage.

A rare but dangerous injury occurs when grease, oil, paraffin, paint or plastic material is injected into the hand as a result of accidental contact with a very high-pressure nozzle. Whether there is only a small local swelling or massive enlargement of the whole hand the affected area needs prompt surgical attention. The first need is to relieve swelling that can so stretch the skin as to jeopardize its survival and the second is to remove as much of the injected matter as possible without delay. The role of the First Aider is to act accordingly; no local treatment is required, only prompt dispatch to medical care.

No breach of the entire thickness of the skin can safely be dismissed by a First Aider as trivial. He should not attempt to explore or probe it but merely apply a dry dressing and send the patient to a doctor. This simple rule has deliberately been emphasized because it is still too often ignored in spite of the large numbers of genuinely trivial injuries that are rightly referred to a doctor.

Definitive treatment

From the surgeon's point of view this can be summed up as inspection, cleansing, exploring, repairing and closing. Severe wounds require blood transfusion and various antibacterial drugs.

The success of treatment depends largely on its being carried out within a few hours of injury in a patient who is fit for what may have to be a lengthy and taxing operation. It is clear that the various means of closure now available offer a good prospect that most civilian and peace-time wounds will heal by first intention if promptly and properly dealt with.

OLDER WOUNDS AND INFECTIONS

In Great Britain most people are acquainted with the signs and symptoms of inflammation and can recognize that a wound has become septic. Their reaction varies from self-treatment at one extreme to consulting a doctor at the other; in between, the advice of First Aiders, chemists and others may be sought. Small septic lesions are so frequent and so often heal whatever is done to them that the possible serious consequences are liable to be ignored. Nevertheless, the First Aider should have reliable guidance in the care of inflammation.

The practice of poulticing and soaking dies hard. Its alleged purpose is to 'bring it to a head'. The fact that suppuration ensues is accepted as confirming the value of these measures and ignores the facts that suppuration is not a process to be encouraged, that suppuration is neither hastened nor delayed by heat, and that pus may appear at the surface only some time after it has formed at greater depth. In the meantime, extensive destruction of important structures may have occurred.

The significance of calor, dolor, tumor, rubor and functio laesa should be as well known to the First Aider as to the medical man; he should also be acquainted with the old surgical adage 'when there is pus, let it out' and be taught the importance of rest in the management of inflammation.

Discomfort, swelling, redness and warmth may subside with rest alone. A cut, scratch or prick followed by these symptoms and signs restricted to the injured area should be dressed and the part put at rest, preferably elevated as well. Hot soaks and poultices may be comforting but sodden tissues heal less well and infection may be added. In the case of a closed lesion such as an incipient boil or abscess, these objections do not apply but there is no virtue in any locally applied medicament. By the time that discomfort has reached the stage of throbbing or has cost the patient a night's sleep, pus has most likely formed and incision should be considered. An inflamed finger that is visibly swollen usually contains pus. The importance of spreading cellulitis, lymphangitis and lymphadenitis is widely recognized.

With sulphonamides, penicillin and other antibiotics so widely prescribed, unused supplies exist in many medicine cupboards and seem to offer the enthusiast a sovereign and 'scientific' remedy. Any such self-treatment is to be condemned. It may limit the spread of infection but cannot be expected to sterilize pus, dissolve dead tissue or reduce the tension that can cause ischaemic necrosis of inflamed tissues. Furthermore, it can induce resistance in germs that were previously sensitive to the drug used and it may also make the patient sensitive and liable to allergic reactions such as rashes, serum sickness and the dramatic and potentially fatal collapse of anaphylaxis.

The First Aider should be urged to refer septic wounds to a doctor without delay. Dressing the wound, no matter how carefully, carries the risk that infection will be added each time the wound is exposed and it does nothing to shorten the course of healing.

Conclusion

Much depends on the surgeon, but his chances of success can only be reduced by dilatory and meddlesome First Aid. If the First Aider can be made to realize the difference between healing by granulation—a slow, painful and possibly crippling process—and healing by first intention, which may mean that one operation and a short period of recovery will see the patient back in harness, much can be done to wean him from the messy applications and makeshift dressings that he so often applies. A rough idea of what can be done and how should arouse his interest and mollify any sense of disappointment at being forbidden many traditional practices.

BANDAGES AND BANDAGING

A bandage has two main purposes—to keep a splint or dressing in place and to apply pressure.

Retentive bandages

Any material that can be made to encircle the part to keep a dressing in place will serve. There is much scope for improvisation and the standard methods using triangular and roller bandages or makeshift substitutes need not be enlarged upon.

Pressure bandages

These are required to stop bleeding and to prevent or reduce swelling. They play a large part in the successful management of grafts and wounds in general but they require considerable care and skill if they are not to be dangerous. The importance of swelling and dusky discoloration beyond the bandage and of pain felt beneath it must be stressed.

Firm, even pressure is best applied by a crape bandage that is fairly well stretched as it is being put on. Even distribution of pressure is aided by applying the bandage over a thick layer of wool. Care must be taken where the bandage overlaps the wool and lies directly on the skin because the edge easily wrinkles and can cause blistering and death of the skin. Elastic bandages containing rubber require especial care because they can constrict dangerously; they should be stretched only slightly when being applied and on the whole they are better avoided. Bandages made entirely of rubber are included in some First Aid kits and require even more care. They are most useful as constrictions on the badly bleeding stumps of amputated limbs or limbs that have to be amputated on the spot. Even so, they are rarely necessary because most traumatic amputations cause remarkably little bleeding.

Bandages used to apply localized pressure to stop bleeding are further considered in Chapter 4.

There should be no hesitation about securing dressings or bandages with adhesive strapping. It is no easy task to apply a bandage neatly and securely at the site of an accident and suitable reinforcement should not be looked upon as a sign of incompetence. A frequent error is to apply elastic strapping at full stretch; if it encircles the limb it will act as a constriction and if it goes only part way round it will pull itself off. The elasticity is intended to allow conformation to uneven surfaces.

ANIMAL BITES

Dogs may produce irregular and complicated but essentially clean-cut wounds by a slashing action. These heal well after cleansing and careful stitching. Much less often a dog will bite out a piece from the lips of a child that tries to kiss it but most often there is little more than grazing and bruising.

Cats' teeth are liable to pierce fingers to the bone and their bites should always be referred to a doctor without delay.

Human bites result in very severe infection because the tissues are badly crushed and at the same time the many potentially pathogenic denizens of the mouth are driven into them. They too require skilled attention without delay.

Domestic and other animals can all inflict more or less serious wounds and all bites require immunizing injections against tetanus.

SHARK BITES

The victim should be brought out of the water as quickly as possible and thereafter kept at rest in the hope that resuscitation equipment can reach him in time. The temptation to rush such a person to hospital in the nearest vehicle must be resisted because the disturbance has sealed the fate of many an exsanguinated victim of this terrible injury. Apart from rapid intravenous infusion of the most readily available liquid any accessible bleeding must be stopped.

SNAKE BITES

The only poisonous snake native to Britain is the adder or viper. Its bite is rarely fatal but a combination of ignorance and fear with the alarming local and general signs has tended to over-emphasize the severity of snake-bite.

The poisons injected by the bite injure the tissues around and cause haemolysis and haemorrhagic exudation. The injured area shows at first the puncture marks of the bite, then oedema and haemorrhagic swelling occur and may spread from the extremity to the root of the limb. Blisters sometimes form. The general effects usually develop within 2 hours or not at all. Giddiness and sweating may go on to nausea, vomiting and prostration. In severe cases the patient is profoundly collapsed and may be unconscious. Children are more likely than adults to be severely affected.

The popular idea of local treatment for snake-bite includes incision followed by sucking the wound or applying a supposed antidote to it. This treatment is to be condemned. Incision has added serious damage by dividing nerves and tendons near the bite; serious infection and sloughing have been promoted by such vigorous maltreatment of the wound.

The only locally applicable treatment that is likely to be of any value is to inject antivenin* and the sooner this is done the better.

The official recommendations for First Aid after snake-bite are:

1. Kill the snake, if possible, and keep it. Handle it only by the tail.
2. Reassure the patient convincingly.
3. Keep the patient at rest. In cases of biting by sea snakes the victim may have no alternative to exerting himself if he is to reach safety and follow the recommended procedures.
4. Wash the bitten surface with plain water, without rubbing.
5. Immobilize the bitten part as for a fracture, and if possible keep it in a dependent position.
6. Administer analgesics such as aspirin, but not morphine.
7. Call a doctor or transfer the patient to hospital together with the dead snake, if available.

Further medical treatment includes 100 mg of hydrocortisone, antibiotics and immunization against tetanus. For the doctor with his bag to hand an antihistamine drug may be given, and if there is time to spare and the materials are available an intravenous infusion of plasma is advisable for the severely shocked person.

In tropical countries various local customs determine the manner of treating snake-bite. Some venoms include rapidly fatal neurotoxins and the only hope of survival lies in preventing the venom from spreading all over the body. Immediate amputation or excision of the bitten

*The viper antivenin available in Britain is useless in this country because it is prepared against a different species of snake.

part can be carried out by the victim. The alternative measure of at once applying a very tight tourniquet above the bite is possible only if someone else is immediately at hand. The tourniquet must be left in place until the part has been amputated.

It is in tropical countries that the use of antihistamine drugs and plasma infusions is most likely to be required because of the distances between hospitals. In general, the victims of snake-bite either die rapidly or recover without painful and destructive methods of treatment, and it is worth remembering that a snake that bites in warning injects less poison than one that bites to kill; the mortality rate from cobra bites is no more than about 50 per cent.

4

BLOOD AND
BLEEDING

BLOOD

Blood is a very complex substance which supplies nourishment to all parts of the body, removes waste products, protects the body against infection and distributes and conserves body heat. To carry out all these functions efficiently there must be a sufficient quantity to reach all the cells in the body. It consists of cells suspended in a liquid called plasma, the cells forming 45 per cent of the total volume.

The total volume of blood is about 70–100ml per kg of bodyweight and is about one-eleventh of the total bodyweight. The volume therefore varies with the size of the person; a large adult has about 6 litres

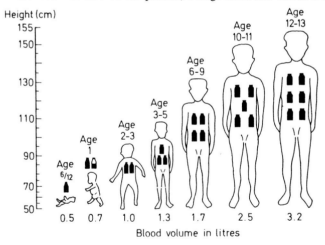

Figure 4.1. Average normal blood volumes in children by age
(From Clark, R. (1959). *Ann. R. Coll. Surg.* **24**, 239)

53

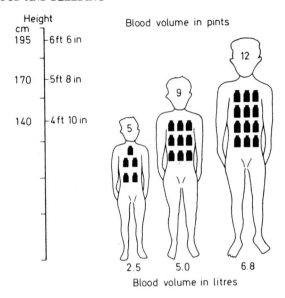

Figure 4.2. Average normal blood volume in adults by height
(From Clarke, R. (1959). *Br. Med. J.* **1**, 125)

of blood, whereas a small baby has about 0.5 litre (*Figures 4.1* and *4.2*).

The cells are developed in the red bone marrow which in the adult is situated mainly in the ribs, sternum and vertebrae. Their life cycle is relatively short—about 6 weeks—and when they die they are removed by the reticulo-endothelial system which consists of cells situated in the liver, spleen, bone marrow and lymph glands.

The cells in the blood are of three kinds—red blood cells, white blood cells or leucocytes, and platelets.

The red blood cells are non-nucleated biconcave discs and normally there are about 5,000,000 per mm^3 of blood. They owe their red colour to the haemoglobin they contain, which is an iron-containing protein for the carriage of oxygen to the tissues.

The white blood cells are colourless nucleated cells. In health there are about 8,000 per mm^3 of blood. They are subdivided into granulocytes and monocytes, of which there are several varieties.

Blood platelets are very small cells about one-eighth the size of a red blood cell and there are about 250,000 per mm^3. They are essential for coagulation or clotting of blood.

Plasma constitutes 55 per cent of the normal circulating blood volume. It contains in solution many salts, mainly sodium chloride, and is 7 per cent protein, of which fibrinogen helps the blood to clot. Glucose is also present in plasma. All these substances are regulated within narrow limits.

Functions

Red blood cells

Red blood cells transport oxygen to all parts of the body by means of the haemoglobin they contain. Deficiency of red blood cells causes anaemia, a condition that deprives the tissues of oxygen.

Oxygen reaches the red cells from inspired air, which is 21 per cent oxygen, by passing through the thin walls of the vessels surrounding the air sacs of the lungs. After circulation round the body the blood returning to the lungs is only 16 per cent oxygen. By the same time carbon dioxide has increased from 0.4 to 4.4 per cent; it is given off on expiration.

White blood cells

These cells have a different function, albeit a very important one, in combating infection. The polymorphonuclear leucocytes are highly active against bacteria, which they engulf and destroy. Lymphocytes have a similar action but are active mainly against chronic infections, such as tuberculosis, and they play a part in immunization processes. In the fight against bacterial invasion many of the white blood cells and bacteria are destroyed and this dead tissue is pus. The white cells increase in number to overcome the infection and may reach 20,000 per mm^3. A form of cancer affecting the white cells is called leukaemia and may raise their number above 100,000 per ml.

White blood cells can also be destroyed by other agents, mainly X-rays and certain drugs, and these are used in the treatment of leukaemia.

Platelets

The platelets are concerned mainly with coagulation or clotting of blood. When a vessel in the body is injured platelets adhere to the site of injury and white cells adhere to the platelets in an attempt to close the breach, but this alone is insufficient. However, the adherent platelets liberate thrombokinase which neutralizes heparin, a normal constituent of plasma, so that calcium and prothrombin, which are present in plasma, form thrombin; this then reacts with soluble fibrinogen to form fibrin, which is the basis of a clot.

Thrombosis is often used to denote the piecemeal accumulation of fibrin and white cells by deposition from moving blood whereas coagulation, or clotting, affects the whole of a stationary mass of blood. Thrombosis can arrest the flow of blood in a vessel and so lead to clotting. Gradually the clot contracts and squeezes out serum, which differs from plasma in that it has lost fibrinogen and cannot clot.

The importance of platelets is that they are essential for the natural process of the arrest of bleeding.

Plasma

The main constituents of plasma are protein, electrolytes, fats and glucose.

The proteins in plasma have three main functions:

1. To help maintain the delicate balance between water inside and outside the capillaries; this is done mainly by albumen. The dropsical swelling that sometimes accompanies kidney disease or malnutrition occurs because the amount of albumin in the blood and consequently its holding power for water is less than it should be.
2. To provide protection against disease, which is the function of the globulins. Immunization against tetanus, for example, causes a change in the aptly named immunoglobulins that confers this protective power upon them.
3. Coagulation, which depends upon the conversion of fibrinogen into fibrin.

Causes of alteration in volume

Bleeding

This is the commonest cause of change in the blood volume. Immediately after bleeding the composition of the blood may show little change, but in a short time the plasma proteins exert their osmotic effect to draw water into the circulation and so dilute the smaller number of red blood cells. The red cell count is therefore lowered, as is the haemoglobin content, even though the red blood cells contain the normal amount of haemoglobin. For the same reason the plasma protein falls. Most of these effects can be overcome by timely and adequate blood transfusion. If transfusion is withheld the deficiency in red blood cells causing a low haemoglobin is the anaemia of trauma.

Burns

In burns there is a loss of red blood cells but proportionately a much larger loss of plasma and consequently of plasma salts and colloids, so that plasma transfusion is more important than blood. Dextran, which is a synthetic colloid made from sugar but resembling protein in its controlling effect on the distribution of water between the capillaries and the surrounding tissues, can also be used to make good the blood volume.

Hartmann's solution resembles normal extracellular fluid in its salt content, so that it adds water to the system without disturbing the balance of salts in the different compartments.

Dehydration

Loss of fluid also reduces the blood volume and is caused by such conditions as sweating, vomiting, diarrhoea, peritonitis and paralytic ileus. The external losses are obvious, but water lost in these conditions is accompanied by severe sodium deficiency which must be made good at the same time as the loss of water.

In peritonitis and paralytic ileus the loss of water is less easily estimated and in peritonitis infection is added to the dehydration. Accurate correction of these and other deficiencies requires measurement of the different constituents, which illustrates the simple effectiveness of the natural methods of control.

Overhydration

The infusion of normal saline or the drinking of large quantities of water is quickly dealt with in the normal subject. When it is absorbed into the bloodstream this raises the capillary pressure, forcing water into the capillary, and also dilutes the plasma proteins; for both these reasons water passes out of the capillaries, but in due course fluid is excreted by the kidneys.

Stagnation

Stasis of blood occurs with bleeding because vasoconstriction narrows the arterioles to such an extent that the blood cannot pass and that in the capillaries beyond stagnates; the venous return to the heart is reduced, causing anoxia, which is greatest in the capillaries of the gut but most easily observed in the bluish discoloration of the lips, ears and fingernails. Fortunately this vasoconstriction is selective, at first, and the brain and heart are spared.

In the early stages the circulation is fully restored by replenishing it with blood, plasma, dextran or even a simple solution of salts but beyond a certain point in the process of response to oligaemia the spasm of the arterioles immediately before the capillaries does not relax when the liquid lost from the circulation has been made good and it may be necessary to give a vasodilator drug. By opening the sluice gates, as it were, this restores the flow through the capillaries, but it also opens up an additional vascular space and in order to fill this it is necessary to give a good deal more blood, or other liquid.

Pressure and flow

It is very easy to take it for granted that if a person has a low blood pressure the last thing one wants to do is to give a vasodilator drug.

Maintaining a high rate of flow through narrow tubes requires a good head of pressure but if the tubes are wide a large flow will result with only a low head of pressure. One may compare the fine but powerful jet that can be squirted from the needle of a syringe with the much larger but less forceful flow, for example, from an enema syringe.

As the amount of blood in circulation falls, the capacity of the blood vessels shrinks and, most important of all, the flow of blood back to the heart becomes so much reduced that its driving force is diminished and the blood pressure falls.

If stagnation continues a condition of widespread but small-scale thrombosis occurs and is known as disseminated intravascular coagulation. Platelets and fibrin in particular become deposited on the walls of the capillaries and as well as being capable of blocking any remaining flow of blood through them this also uses up the clotting power of the blood and causes the patient to bleed, a condition known as consumption coagulopathy.

Fortunately, this grave state of affairs is very rare but the whole sequence of events emphasizes the vital importance of doing all that is possible to curtail bleeding, avoid disturbance and enable the patient to receive appropriately skilled treatment as soon as possible.

Circulation

The heart acts as a pump forcing the blood round the body. Blood from the right side of the heart is pumped into the lungs via the pulmonary arteries and after oxygenation returns to the heart via the pulmonary veins and is ejected through the aortic valve into the aorta.

The *rate* of the heart beat is controlled mainly by the vagus nerve from the brain. It has an inhibitory effect on the heart when stimulated but by variations in the inhibitory tone of the nerve the heart rate may slow or accelerate. The heart is also, but to a lesser extent, under the influence of the sympathetic nervous system, stimulation of which causes the heart to accelerate, as occurs when a subject is frightened or undergoes exercise. Conversely an emotional upset stimulates the vagus nerve and may so slow the heart as to cause fainting in severe cases. The heart rate is also affected by certain reflexes arising from receptors on the aorta, the carotid arteries and the great veins to the heart.

The carotid and aortic bodies are chemoreceptors and are affected by the amount of carbon dioxide and oxygen in the blood. Anoxia or excess carbon dioxide increases the heart rate and acidifies the blood. Sinuses on the carotid, aorta and great veins are affected by pressure. As the pressure in aortic or carotid arteries rises so the heart rate slows but if the pressure rises in the great veins the vagus nerve is reflexly depressed and the heart rate accelerates.

Temperature also affects the heart rate, a rise producing quickening of the rate by stimulation of the sino-auricular node which is the termination of the right vagus nerve in the heart.

The body temperature is accurately controlled by a balance between heat production and heat loss. Heat is produced, mainly, by muscle activity and lost by vaporization, convention and conduction. The vascularity of the skin, the activity of sweat glands, pulmonary ventilation, the activity of muscles and secreting glands are under the control of the nervous system and these nerve centres are affected by the temperature of the blood, so that increases in temperature cause vasodilatation and sweating to reduce the temperature.

The adrenal medulla and thyroid gland, also, when stimulated reflexly raise the metabolic rate and so heat production.

Cardiac output

At each heart beat approximately 100 ml of blood are injected into aorta; this is the stroke volume but the output is more usually expressed as the minute volume and is between 5 and 6 litres a minute from each ventricle, that from the right side going to the lungs and that from the left to the systemic circulation via the aorta.

With each injection of blood the arterial column of blood moves onwards and distends the arterial wall. It is this distension which gives rise to the pulse wave and it is not related to the blood flow rate.

The rate of blood flow is inversely proportional to the cross section of the vascular bed of the part and in the capillaries is only about $\frac{1}{2000}$ of that in the aorta. The flow in the aorta is nearly 1 metre/second. The slowing down of the rate of flow is due to the large arteries dividing into smaller arteries, arterioles and capillaries and then coalescing to form venules, veins and the great veins which run back to the right side of the heart. The final rate of flow in the great veins is much slower than in the aorta. Veins in the neck can sometimes be seen to pulsate; this is partly an effect of the respiratory pulse and partly of back flow from the heart along the intervening valveless veins. The output of the heart depends on the venous return, the force and frequency of the heart beat.

Return of venous blood

The return of venous blood to the heart is helped by muscular contractions that squeeze the blood along the veins, by the sucking effect of the act of breathing on the thin-walled veins in the chest and by the pressure in the capillaries pushing the blood along.

Capillary and venous tone vary and when the vessels constrict the rate of blood flow is increased, for when dilated the capillaries can hold a large quantity of blood which does not reach the veins. In bleeding the constriction of the veins is one of the natural ways the body has of maintaining an adequate venous return.

Force of the heart beat

The force depends on the degree of filling of the heart. The greater the distension of the ventricles the greater the force with which it contracts. When the blood volume is low the heart becomes underfilled and consequently the force of the beat is less.

Diminished oxygen supply impairs nutrition and when the heart muscle is affected in this way the force of its beat is reduced.

Distribution of blood

This varies through a fairly wide range but the kidneys receive about 1 litre and of the remainder 2—3 litres go to the abdominal viscera and 1.5—2.0 litres to the muscles, brain, coronary arteries and the skin. Skin and muscle show the greatest variation, depending on the degree of vasoconstriction in the skin and the degree of activity of the muscle. In vigorous activity the flow to the muscles is greatly increased.

Blood pressure

The product of the cardiac output and the peripheral resistance is the blood pressure. As the ventricle contracts it has to increase the pressure within it sufficiently to open the aortic valve against the pressure in the aorta to eject the blood it contains; this is the systolic pressure and is normally about 120 mmHg.

The pressure within the ventricle after the ejection phase, when the ventricle is relaxed, known as the diastolic pressure, is much lower, normally about 70 mmHg. The blood pressure is therefore expressed as 120/70 mmHg and variations depend on the cardiac output and the peripheral resistance.

Peripheral resistance

This is under the control of the vasomotor centre in the brain and controlling impulses are conducted by the sympathetic nerve fibres from the spinal cord to the arteries and particularly to the arterioles. Central stimulation causes capillary constriction and this affects particularly the intestine and skin; hence the well-known pallor and coolness caused by bleeding.

If, however, the spinal cord is transected in the neck, because of a fractured cervical vertebra, the sympathetic nerve fibres are cut off from the brain and a marked capillary dilatation results with a consequent fall in blood pressure, which is why the term 'spinal shock' is applied to this clinical state. Gradually the local reflexes take over and the blood pressure returns to normal but this does not necessarily mean that the spinal cord is recovering.

Later in life as the arteries harden because of arteriosclerosis the peripheral resistance is increased so that older people tend to have a raised blood pressure to overcome the resistance in the more rigid arterioles.

Ischaemia

If the blood supply to a mass of tissue is cut off, eventually that tissue will die. This is seen most characteristically in coronary thrombosis, where the artery is occluded. The area affected is known as an infarct, intense pain follows and the heart muscle functions less efficiently so the cardiac output and the blood pressure fall. If the patient survives then the area of muscle dies and forms a scar.

If the blood supply to the kidneys is inadequate, then the kidneys produce a substance called renin, which in combination with the plasma protein forms angiotonin. This leads to hypertension due to vasoconstriction, which affects the kidney function by diminishing its blood supply and may eventually lead to uraemia and death. Hence the importance of restoring the blood volume to normal. A blood pressure of 50 mmHg for more than 4 hours usually stops the excretion of urine, which is known as anuria, in which case an artificial kidney can be used until either the patient's own kidneys recover or are replaced by a transplanted one.

Blood groups

Although the first experiments with animals were carried out some 200 years ago the administration of one person's blood to another became a practicable procedure only when Landsteiner identified the four main blood groups early in the present century and called them O, A, B and AB. Unless the donor's blood is accurately matched with the recipient's, substances in the plasma of one will destroy the cells of the other. Group O blood has been called the universal donor because its plasma is free of substances (agglutinins) that damage the cells of blood in the other three groups. In fact, as more and more subgroups have been recognized it has become increasingly important to match blood accurately. If this is not done there is the danger that if a recipient receives a 'strange' factor in someone else's blood his own blood will undergo changes that would lead to the destruction of a further quantity of blood containing the now familiar factor. The most important of these is the rhesus factor, which was identified over 40 years ago as the explanation for the early death of some babies with severe jaundice and the survival as lame brains of others that had been deeply jaundiced at birth.

The explanation is that if a woman with rhesus negative blood has a husband who is rhesus positive her baby is likely to be rhesus positive. The positive factor in her baby's blood is 'strange' to the mother's blood, which acquires the power to destroy the red cells in her baby's.

This destructive power increases with each succeeding rhesus positive child so that whereas the first may survive without serious damage, later infants are exposed to increasing risk of fatal consequences of the incompatibility of their blood with that of their mother.

BLEEDING

By bleeding is meant loss of blood from the circulation, not necessarily from the body. If the skin surface is broken then bleeding is obvious; if, however, the skin is not broken bleeding can still occur but will be less obvious and its cause and site may be difficult to determine.

The causes of bleeding are trauma, disease and drugs.

Trauma

Any injury to the body will cause bleeding of some degree. If the injury is slight and the skin not broken some capillaries will be damaged causing very little bleeding into the subcutaneous tissues and forming a bruise, which undergoes the characteristic colour changes.

More severe injury produces greater bleeding and swelling. This swelling is called a haematoma and can be small or very extensive. The small haematoma resolves quite quickly but the large one may take many weeks to be absorbed. The commonest large haematomata are seen around closed fractures, such as fractures of the pelvis or femur, and may be of sufficient extent to require blood transfusion, for though the blood has not been lost from the body it has been lost from the circulation and may amount to several litres.

Injuries of the joints may be associated with bleeding into or around the joint. Bleeding occurs around a joint when there has been a sprain or the more serious tearing of the enveloping tissues, such as accompanies dislocation. Bleeding which occurs into a joint when its capsule is intact is known as haemarthrosis, and is frequently caused by a fracture into a joint.

Bleeding into the tissues is such a familiar occurrence that it is in most cases rightly dismissed as 'just a bruise', but ambulancemen, nurses and doctors are only too well aware of a much more serious sort, so serious, indeed, that the amount of blood lost from circulation may endanger the patient's life.

In open wounds the skin is broken and blood escapes. The degree of bleeding depends not only on the nature of the wound, but the site and the vessels involved.

A simple cut in the skin produces little bleeding as only skin capillaries have been divided. Deeper cuts may involve arteries and bleeding may be severe, the blood spurting out with each heart beat.

At other times a large vein rather than an artery may be cut and bleeding is under less pressure and is continuous, not spurting, and darker in colour. But in most serious wounds arteries and veins are cut and there is a mixture of arterial and venous blood.

In a contused or tearing type of wound the bleeding tends to be less because the injury causes more contraction and retraction of the vessels (*see* Natural arrest of bleeding). Some parts of the body are more vascular than others, such as the hands and face so that size for size, wounds in these areas bleed more.

Bleeding from bones is more continuous than from soft tissues because the vessels are in bony canals and cannot retract and contract as in soft tissues.

Internal organs such as the liver and spleen, whether subjected to blunt trauma or incised wounds from stabbing, bleed very freely for they have a very rich blood supply.

Ulceration is the result of a breach of continuity of tissue which fails to heal by primary union. The failure to heal is usually due to an infection but may be due to an inadequate blood supply, as in a varicose ulcer, or to the growth of abnormal tissue, as in cancer.

Varicose ulcers only occur in areas which are affected by varicose veins, most commonly in the legs, but may occur in the oesophagus or rectum. Veins become varicose when the valves in the veins become inadequate, which may be due to obstruction or over-distension. When the valves are inadequate the return of blood to the heart is less efficient due to hydrostatic pressure so that the skin contains more venous blood and becomes less well nourished and may break down and form an ulcer. Should the varicose vein rupture due to some minor injury then severe bleeding occurs.

Neoplasms are new growths of tissue. The innocent variety sometimes cause bleeding, as in 'polyps' of the intestinal wall. The malignant variety, or 'cancers', frequently cause bleeding because of their rapid growth. Such bleeding is usually continuous and only serious because it occurs over a long period, producing anaemia.

Disease

The notable diseases which cause bleeding are uncommon but serious. They are: haemophilia, purpura and scurvy and liver diseases.

Haemophilia

This is one of the bleeding diseases due to a deficiency of a factor—in this case Factor VIII—from the plasma. The coagulation time is greatly prolonged, even though all the normal constituents necessary for coagulation are present in the blood. The disease is an inherited anomaly transmitted by females, who do not suffer from the disease, to males who may show signs of the disease. Continuous bleeding which becomes severe because it persists for so long may follow the most trivial injury. Most haemophiliacs know they have the disease and usually carry a card or 'Medic-alert' disc indicating that they are haemophiliacs and where they normally receive treatment.

The treatment for these patients is to supply the missing factor as a concentrate, but more easily available in an emergency is fresh frozen plasma or cryoprecipitate, the latter being an excellent haemostatic agent.

Purpura

In this disease bleeding can occur spontaneously without injury and is due to a deficiency in platelets. In many cases the cause of the deficiency is unknown but can be produced by deep X-ray therapy or misuse of drugs, causing pernicious anaemia or aplastic anaemia.

It can be treated by platelet-rich plasma or platelet concentrates, at least temporarily, but the cause of deficiency in platelets must also be treated.

Scurvy

Once a common disease, scurvy is now very rare and is due to a deficiency of vitamin C. It causes prolonged bleeding time but the clotting time is normal. It is still seen among people who live at near-starvation level. Fractures and wounds fail to heal and blood clots fail to organize so that excessive bleeding follows injury, but may occur spontaneously from the gums, bladder and bowel.

The treatment is a diet of fresh fruit and vegetables, or taking pills containing ascorbic acid.

Lack of vitamin K

Vitamin K is found in most normal foodstuffs and so is rarely absent from the diet. It is essential for the formation of plasma prothrombin.

It may be deficient in liver diseases, such as obstructive jaundice and cirrhosis of the liver, and result in the failure of prothrombin formation, so that injury or operation may cause excessive bleeding.

The deficiency of vitamin K can be made good by injecting vitamin K intramuscularly.

Drugs

Certain drugs have an anticoagulant effect and are given to patients to avoid thrombosis, or intravascular clotting, particularly in the aged bed-ridden, who are prone to thrombosis. They have also been used in the treatment of coronary thrombosis.

Heparin is normally present in the body, being secreted by the mast cells and is responsible for the normal fluidity of the blood. Sometimes heparin is used as an anticoagulant in patients who have had a thrombosis to prevent the thrombus spreading to the pulmonary artery and causing obstruction of the blood flow to the lungs.

Dicoumarin and warfarin have a similar action by reducing the prothrombin concentration and the risk of thrombosis.

In old people in hospital these drugs are now frequently given in controlled doses to prevent thrombosis occurring. Such patients are always given a card stating that they are on these drugs so that should they start bleeding the correct treatment of giving vitamin K can be started at once.

Natural arrest of bleeding

Pressure

When bleeding occurs under intact skin, as in a bruise, the pressure increases sufficiently to stop or slow the bleeding for coagulation to occur.

In the abdomen, bleeding does not produce the same degree of pressure because the abdominal wall is distensible and can accommodate considerable quantities of blood before any significant pressure develops.

The brain is soft and deformable and because the skull is hard bleeding within the skull can occur only be displacing the brain; this affects the vital centres, causing death before sufficient pressure has developed to arrest bleeding. Hence the urgency of diagnosing and relieving intracranial bleeding.

Retraction and contraction

All vessels contain muscle and elastic tissue so that they can contract or dilate. This is especially so in large arteries but much less so in the veins. Their contractility is under nervous control exerted by the vaso-motor centre in the brain. When vessels are stimulated, as by injury, they contract and retract and this helps to narrow the lumen so aiding coagulation.

Sometimes this contraction and retraction is so intense, especially after tearing injuries against incised wounds, that bleeding from very large arteries may be arrested very quickly with little loss of blood although a large loss would be expected. This applies particularly in the young patient who has healthy arteries. As age advances the arteries become more rigid from loss of their elastic tissue and may in some cases become calcified so that neither retraction nor contraction can occur, bleeding is persistent and coagulation delayed.

Depletion of the blood supply

As bleeding continues so the blood volume diminishes and this will in time lower the blood pressure for the heart can only eject what it receives. The fall in blood pressure produces a less forceful ejection of blood from the cut vessels, which allows coagulation to occur more readily and seal off the end of the vessel.

Coagulation

This has been described above. It is a very important process and essential for the natural arrest of bleeding.

Rest

This reduces the blood pressure and so reduces the force and flow of blood and thereby reduces the bleeding after injury, so aiding coagu-lation. Hence the importance of laying down an injured patient. This rest can be further assisted in the case of limb injuries by elevating the injured limb so reducing the pressure and flow rate.

Effects on circulation

Bleeding produces a train of events in the body. Where there has been a loss of less than 10 per cent of the blood volume only small changes occur. The heart rate may increase and the blood pressure fall slightly but these soon cease as restoration of the blood volume occurs because extracellular fluid is drawn into the vessels by the osmotic pressure of the plasma proteins, and red blood cells are regenerated from the bone marrow. We see this state of affairs frequently in blood donors, who give approximately 10 per cent of their blood volume without any significant, noticeable changes.

When 20–30 per cent is lost more appreciable changes occur. The blood pressure falls due to less venous return and the heart rate quickens. There is a selective vasoconstriction caused by hormones secreted by the adrenal gland, which affects primarily the skin and muscles and the effect of the hormones of the pituitary gland causes vasoconstriction of the kidneys, thus conserving fluid.

Sodium is retained in the plasma, which becomes further diluted to make up the loss of circulating volume. As bleeding continues the plasma proteins become more diluted and lose their osmotic pressure effect. Vasoconstriction is no longer selective as bleeding progresses and becomes generalized so that all the tissues suffer from anoxia. This affects dangerously the brain, the heart and the lungs. The heart is affected because the fall in blood pressure reduces the coronary flow, which is further reduced by vasoconstriction so that the heart muscle becomes ischaemic and unable to function properly; this further reduces the cardiac output.

The anoxia of the brain gradually increases and unconsciousness may result.

Vasoconstriction affects the intestinal arterioles and produces pooling of blood in the capillaries, which at one time was thought to be the cause of shock. This pooling reduces the circulatory blood volume even further. Vasoconstrictor drugs are therefore not indicated and neither are vasodilator drugs unless the blood volume can be restored adequately and quickly enough.

Acidosis develops and this too needs correction with sodium bicarbonate or a similar buffer solution.

Treatment of bleeding and its effects

Local pressure

In most instances bleeding from open wounds can be controlled by direct pressure on the wound. The effect of this is that the tissues are pressed against some resistant tissue; in the limbs this is usually bone. Similarly all scalp bleeding can be controlled by direct pressure against the skull, so that all that is required is a pad of dressing and a firm bandage.

In large, open, deep wounds direct pressure on the surface of the wound may be inadequate. In these cases the wound should be packed with sterile dressing and then the covering dressing and bandage firmly applied. By this method even large wounds in the groin with bleeding from the femoral artery can be controlled (*Figure 4.3*).

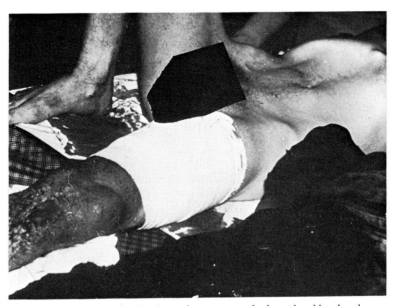

Figure 4.3. A wound of the femoral artery properly dressed and bandaged

The rule that with external bleeding one should press where the blood is coming from has two exceptions, but they are fortunately rare. One is bleeding from the brain or from within the skull when the brain is visible in the wound and the other is bleeding either from or near to an injured eye. In both these cases, the danger of applying pressure to such delicate structures outweighs the danger of continued bleeding. One can only apply a firm, bulky dressing, elevate the part, if possible, keep the patient at rest and arrange for him to receive skilled help as soon as possible.

In closed wounds of the limb such as occur with fractures, bleeding is naturally arrested when the tension in the tissues from extravasated blood is high enough to arrest the arterial bleeding. This is associated with much swelling. The process may be aided by a firm crape bandage to increase pressure, splinting to minimize further trauma, and elevation to reduce the blood flow.

Should the bleeding continue in open wounds and come through the dressing, the primary dressing should not be removed for this may restart bleeding from many points at which it has already been arrested. It is easy to apply a further bandage firmly over a thick layer of wool to help to increase the local pressure.

Recurrent bleeding may occur in any wound and is usually due to interference with the dressing or to the ligature coming off a vessel after an operation. Pressure should be reapplied until the vessel can be properly ligated. Where large vessels are likely to be involved adequate blood for transfusion should be in readiness before surgery commences.

Reactionary bleeding occurs most frequently from smaller vessels when the blood pressure has been restored by transfusion. Ligation of the vessels may be necessary but usually a pressure dressing is all that is required.

Secondary bleeding occurs 7–10 days after wounding and is nearly always the result of infection. The infection acts on the clot sealing the vessel and destroys it. Such bleeding is difficult to control for the tissues are friable.

The head, chest and abdomen

Apart from skin and scalp wounds, bleeding from the head and from the chest and abdomen cannot be controlled by local pressure.

Bleeding from fractures of the skull or from inside the skull, or from within the chest, can only be controlled surgically.

Any external wound in these areas should be covered with a sterile dressing to counter infection and the patient transferred to hospital as quickly as possible.

Bleeding from within the abdomen cannot be controlled except by an operation. If there is a large wound packing the wound is usually ineffective because the abdomen is distensible and pressure cannot be maintained. The only satisfactory treatment is a sterile cover and quick despatch to hospital, where blood can be grouped and cross-matched and the bleeding points found and ligated.

The pelvis

Some of the most severe bleeding of all can occur from a fracture of the pelvis when a large blood vessel is torn. An inflatable splint, shaped like a pair of trousers has been available in recent years and this has been used in such cases with evident benefit. It is not important for the First Aider if the explanation is that the benefit may owe more to augmenting the amount of blood in circulation by squeezing it out of the lower limbs than to any effect on the bleeding point or area but it is important to remember that even if such an appliance is available it requires great care and much assistance to apply it both safely and effectively to a person with multiple injuries.

'Pressure points'

The use of various 'pressure points' for the control of major bleeding from various parts of the body has long been familiar to all First Aiders. The object is to apply direct manual pressure over the main artery proximal to the bleeding point.

In some cases it is the only method available because local pressure dressings and bandages cannot be applied adequately. The main areas where this is so are in the neck, the armpit (or axilla) and the groin. Severe bleeding from such areas may demand direct manual pressure over the artery proximal to the wound, as well as over the wound itself.

The method is limited by the difficulty of maintaining adequate pressure for any length of time, the difficulty of keeping the pressure applied while the patient is being transferred to ambulance and later into hospital, and also it does not control bleeding from collateral vessels. If there are many casualties it ties one First Aider completely to one patient at the expense of other patients. So, as far as possible manual pressure over pressure points should be avoided. It can be helpful, if an assistant is available, to apply pressure on an artery while a dressing is being applied.

Constriction

As a First Aid measure, tourniquets for the control of bleeding are undesirable because of the many hazards involved and it usually happens that in the sort of case in which a tourniquet can be used a safer or more effective method is practicable.

The main disadvantages of a tourniquet are:

1. The constriction is painful in a conscious patient and pain increases restlessness.

2. If applied too tightly it may injure tissues unaffected by the injury, particularly nerves if they be close to bone.

3. If applied too loosely it obstructs the veins but not the arteries; this increases the bleeding because none of the blood passing the tourniquet can return to the general circulation and the veins beyond quickly become distended and the limb turns blue. Blood is just pumped out of the wound often under pressure nearly equal to arterial pressure, whereas if no tourniquet were used bleeding would continue but some would return to the general circulation by way of patent veins. The pressure that is required is on the injured vessels only.

4. It may be applied and forgotton. It might seem that such an accident could never happen but it does from time to time and is a tragedy, for amputation may be necessary later. It is most likely to occur when many persons have been injured. The tourniquet is applied to one patient and the attendant then goes to another patient; in the meantime the first patient is moved to a First Aid post or hospital and because he is not bleeding the danger of his condition goes unrecognized, particularly if the tourniquet is applied on the proximal part of the limb and covered with clothes.

Anyone applying a tourniquet is therefore morally bound to stay with the patient, to release it for 5 minutes in every 20 minutes and to see that it is finally removed in 2 hours. This is a waste of manpower and time when the bleeding can nearly always be controlled by other means.

In general there is no place for the use of the tourniquet in First Aid practice except for treatment of bleeding amputation stumps (which are very rare) and severe crush injuries of limbs of more than 4 hours' duration (*see* Chapter 3).

Dressings

These are adequate when they control the bleeding, are comfortable and will not come off or come loose when the patient is moved. Although it is desirable that they should look tidy this is not the most important point.

The application of a dressing that is firm enough to stanch bleeding but not so tight that it will act as a venous tourniquet and cause congestion and swelling of the limb beyond it calls for both experience and skill. However, it is easy to teach by demonstration what happens when a bandage is too tight. Applying an adequate, firm bandage is much easier with a crape, kling or crinx bandage than with an ordinary cotton one because they conform to the contour of the dressing and the limb, but they are more expensive.

Rest

This is essential for an injured patient because anxiety due to pain or general restlessness increases the blood pressure and so the bleeding. The patient should be lain down and reassured; if surgical treatment is likely to be long-delayed pain-relieving injections intravenously in small doses are permissible, but it is worth mentioning that in most cases persons complaining of pain are more frightened than injured and that the severely injured are often silent and uncomplaining. Thus, in case of multiple casualties rescuers should not at once go to the aid of the plaintive and vociferous, but survey the scene and decide for themselves who needs to have what done first.

With limb injuries, elevation of the limb should be carried out, if possible, because this lowers the blood pressure and assists the venous return. To do this it may be necessary to dress the wound and splint the limb, so that it is comfortable, before elevation. Reassurance helps the patient to rest quietly and an inflatable splint makes it all much easier although it does not always stop the bleeding.

Drinking

Although the natural way of maintaining the body's water supply is by drinking, and although some patients will complain insistently of thirst because they have lost more than 10—15 per cent of their blood, drinking can lead to vomiting and the risk of inhaling the vomitus. Moistening the lips with a wet swab helps to add to their comfort but patients with a thirst are usually in need of intravenous infusion.

Intravenous infusions

When more than a donation or two of blood has been lost it is desirable that the loss be made good by the administration of blood when this is possible. Among the limiting factors is the fact that the group O rhesus negative blood that can safely be given without preliminary grouping and matching is too scarce to be carried by emergency teams as a matter of course. Fortunately there are few occasions when blood and blood alone will meet a patient's requirements.

Plasma can be given if available, but usually this is so only in hospital. It also has the disadvantages that the dried plasma has first to be mixed with and dissolved in sterile water and that plasma does not run freely through fine tubes.

The next most satisfactory is either dextran which, having a large molecule that does not pass readily through the vessel wall, acts as a plasma expander by increasing the osmotic pressure and drawing in extracellular fluid, or Hartmann's solution, or normal saline. These latter two are easily available, readily sterilized and cheap.

But putting up an intravenous infusion at the site of an accident, where First Aid is carried out, carries with it the risk of infection from lack of sterility in the process.

Haemostatic agents

Although there is a wide range of substances that can be applied to a wound, or be given by mouth, or by injection in order to stop bleeding, these are not suitable for First Aid.

Gelatin sponge, fibrin foam or thrombin topical can be applied to large areas of capillary oozing to promote coagulation.

Thomboral can be given orally for gastro-intestinal bleeding and haemoplastin and vitamin K can be given by injection for the control of bleeding, vitamin K being especially useful to counteract bleeding due to anticoagulant therapy.

Infusion of fresh whole blood, platelet-rich plasma or platelet concentrates have powerful haemostatic effects in patients with platelet deficiency diseases.

Assessment of blood loss

Circulatory patterns

Severe exsanguination is easily recognizable for the patient has a marked fall in blood pressure, which may not be recordable, a weak, rapid pulse up to 150–200/minute, ashen grey facies with blanched extremities and a cold sweating skin due to vasoconstriction, which is another manifestation of nervous activity. The patient becomes garrulous and restless, may vomit and even become unconscious with deep sighing respiration. It is important to be aware that in many respects the patient's condition resembles the restless confusion that sometimes follows head injury and that when there are clear signs that the head has been injured the First Aider should look also for these other causes of restlessness.

There are several stages between severe exsanguination and normal which should be recognized so that one can have some indication of the degree of urgency.

Tachycardia and hypotension

A blood donor gives nearly 0.5 litre of blood without any noticeable change; this is about 10 per cent of his blood volume. More than 10 per cent blood loss causes an increase in the pulse rate (tachycardia) and if this is associated with a normal blood pressure the loss is not more than 20 per cent of the blood volume. If, however, it is associated with a falling blood pressure and pale, cool extremities, then the loss is nearer 30 per cent. This is a fairly critical point because although the patient may appear fairly fit only a little further loss may produce profound collapse. Such a collapse may be precipitated by injudicious handling, anaesthesia, the manipulation of a fracture, or a long ambulance journey. This stage is frequently termed 'latent shock' and is an important state to recognize.

It must, however, be appreciated that the First Aider will be going to the patient's aid soon after injury and that most of the bleeding will occur afterwards into the tissues and the dressings, so that the picture is constantly changing with some overlap of the various stages and signs. The greater the speed of blood loss the quicker will be the collapse for the body has no time to make good the blood volume which it does when the same amount is lost over a longer period.

The circulatory pattern is not therefore a reliable guide to the patient's blood loss but it is helpful especially when assessed with the patient's other signs of injury and the number and size of the wounds, and whether they are closed or open.

The size of the wound

The size of the wound in closed injuries is indicated roughly by the volume of swelling, which is useful only for confirming, not for predicting the order of loss. In open wounds the size refers to the volume of tissue damaged, not just the superficial part of the wound that is visible.

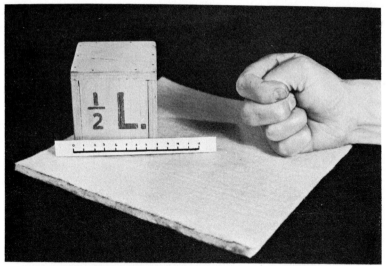

Figure 4.4. A cube, a fist and a piece of felt each equivalent approximately to 1 pint
(From Clarke, R. *et al.* (1955). *Lancet* **1,** 629)

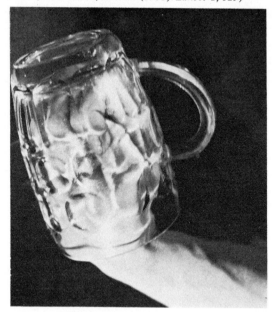

Figure 4.5. A fist in a pint tankard

77

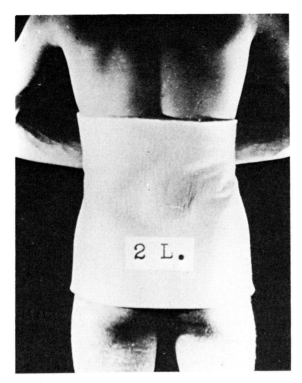

Figure 4.6. A piece of felt 2 litres in volume wrapped round the trunk

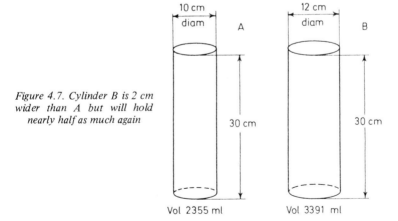

Figure 4.7. Cylinder B is 2 cm wider than A but will hold nearly half as much again

Closed wounds

First of all it is well to be familiar with the volume of certain common objects. For example, a tennis ball has a volume of 0.25 litre.

An adult's fist has a volume of approximately 0.5 litre (*Figure 4.4*) and fits into a pint mug (*Figure 4.5*). A piece of felt 30 X 17 X 1 cm is equal to 0.5 litre and being only 1 cm thick it would not make much difference to the visible size if wrapped round a forearm.

Similarly a piece of felt 70 X 30 X 1 cm has a volume of 2 litres but when wrapped round the waist (*Figure 4.6*) it does not make much difference to the contours. The important point is that it is not just the thickness of the swelling that matters but the area that it occupies. Using a cylinder as an example this is more obvious. *Figure 4.7* shows 2 cylinders. Cylinder A is 30 cm long and 5 cm in radius. The volume

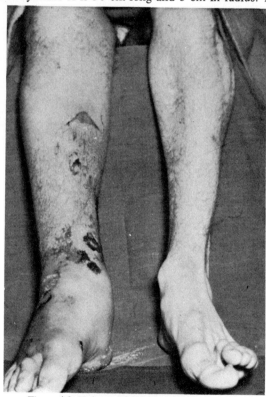

Figure 4.8. Volume of right leg 1 litre more than left following closed fracture of tibia
(Reproduced by courtesy of *Br. J. clin. Pract.* (1956). **10**)

is given by $\pi r^2 \times l$ where r = radius and l = length. The volume therefore is $\pi \times 25 \times 30 = 2,355$ ml. Cylinder B is 30 cm long and has a radius of 6 cm. Its volume therefore is $\pi \times 36 \times 30 = 3,391$ ml. The difference is 1,036 ml so that for an increase in diameter of only 2 cm, the cylinder can contain an extra litre.

In the same way, with swollen limbs it is the volume increase which is important. *Figure 4.8* shows a right leg with a closed fracture of the tibia 1 litre greater in volume than the left. Similarly *Figure 4.9* shows a closed fracture of the femur with swelling equal to 1 litre. The swelling appears wider but this is possibly because the limb is shortened and one should remember that deformity may mask swelling.

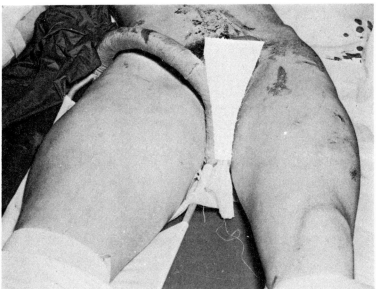

Figure 4.9. Deformed thigh with 1 litre swelling (shortening has allowed greater lateral expansion)

At hospital further information is obtained by X-ray examination, which gives a clue to the degree of bony damage. A comminuted fracture of the tibia may lose 2 litres of blood whereas a simple oblique fracture only 0.5 litre. Therefore when ascertaining the injury and the swelling the degree of violence is an important consideration.

Open wounds

In the case of an open wound bleeding is obvious, but some attempt must be made to assess how much is lost at the scene of the accident, on the clothes and on the stretcher. This is not easy because different materials have different absorptive properties.

The use of the hand in the estimation of bleeding needs to be clearly understood, particularly when one is dealing with patients of unusual size. *Figures 4.1* and *4.2* show that the blood volume of normal individuals ranges from 0.5 litre at birth to 6 or 7 litres in a very tall man. Thus, if one expresses the size of the wound in terms of the size of an adult's hand a 'one-hand wound' would have a negligible effect on a very large person but would exsanguinate a child. If, however, one uses the patient's own hand this represents a fairly constant proportion—about 10 per cent of the blood volume.

Abdominal and pelvic injuries

In abdominal and pelvic injuries the bleeding is internal and hidden and swelling is rarely seen so the assessment of oligaemic shock depends largely on the circulatory pattern. Greater difficulty is experienced when an abdominal or pelvic injury is associated with an obvious major limb injury for only by accurate assessment of the limb injury can any approximation of the degree of oligaemia due to the abdominal injury be made. If the signs of oligaemia are out of all proportion to the limb injury then the abdominal injury may account for the rest. A severe fracture of the pelvis may lose as much as 3 litres of blood quite quickly and may lose up to 10 litres if transfusion keeps the patient alive and allows bleeding to continue. This waste is negligible when it is set against the saving of life and allows for early operation on a fit patient.

Estimation of plasma and red cell volumes

Although the First Aider has to be content with simple observations he should not underestimate the value of an informed understanding of the significance of the patient's condition in the light of a general idea of the degree and extent of violence to which he has been subjected. Our understanding in this respect owes a great deal to the careful measurement of blood lost from the body, the amount of blood still in circulation and swelling of limbs in relation to the patient's condition at the time.

The measurement of blood volume depends upon the intravenous injection of a precisely known volume of an identifiable substance. This may be a dye—Evans blue—or for greater accuracy albumen labelled with radioactive iodine (^{131}I) or alternatively red cells labelled with radiochromium (^{51}Cr) which is allowed to circulate for long enough to become evenly mixed with the blood. Its concentration in the blood is then measured accurately and the volume of blood required to produce that degree of dilution is easily calculated. In practice one measures the volume of either the plasma or the red cells and derives the blood volume from this by measuring the proportion of cells in a given volume of blood. This is known as the packed cell volume or haematocrit; the cells normally provide 40–45 per cent of the total volume.

These methods are accurate to within about 10 per cent in normal persons but much less accurate in the severely oligaemic patient because of inadequate mixing of the dye or isotopes.

Replenishment of the blood volume

Blood transfusion is the method of choice for blood loss, because it supplies red blood cells, plasma and proteins.

Blood in liquid form can be stored for up to a month after which time the red cells degenerate and the blood is no longer either safe or effective as a carrier of oxygen. Blood can be stored indefinitely in freeze-dried form; this is of particular value for keeping rare or otherwise special types of blood for reference purposes but in the process of preparation and reconstitution the blood is damaged to an extent that reduces its effectiveness by 20–30 per cent. However, when blood is no longer safe for intravenous use it is used as a source of constituents that do not deteriorate with keeping and have a therapeutic value in special cases.

The object of blood transfusion is to replace the amount of blood lost as soon as possible and to keep pace with any continuing loss until bleeding has been controlled. This will necessitate continuing the transfusion after any operation for the control of bleeding because blood continues for many hours to be lost by general oozing from the operation area, particularly where there are fractures, because it is not possible to control the bleeding from fractured bone ends.

Some idea of the amount and duration of continuing bleeding can be gained from the fact that if it takes 5 litres of blood to resuscitate a casualty it will take another 5 litres to carry him through whatever operations are required and a further litre or two to make good further loss. Men wounded in battle and picked up within minutes of being wounded have been found to require an average of about 8 litres of blood. Sometimes large amounts of blood are required and to cope with the demand it may be necessary to have more than one intravenous infusion of blood going at any one time. Arterial transfusions have been tried, but have not proved more successful than adequate intravenous transfusions and they are less easy to perform.

Plasma transfusions are used mainly in treating burns but plasma offers a good substitute for blood when blood is not available or as a preliminary transfusion while awaiting the full grouping and cross-matching of blood. However, because it does not run easily it is not a satisfactory infusate for use during transport of a casualty. Unlike blood it can be stored for years.

The hazards of blood transfusions are incompatibility, infection, giving too much too quickly and so overloading the heart, and in the confusion of dealing with mass casualties giving blood to the wrong patient; with proper precautions these hazards are uncommon.

Plasma and blood also carry the risk of causing jaundice though this is much less common now.

Hypothermia

Certain animals hibernate during the winter, during which time they take no food and appear to be in a deep sleep. Their body temperature falls and their breathing is very shallow because their body requirements are so low that they do not require much oxygen.

If the temperature of the body is raised by restlessness, or artificially, the demands for oxygen are increased and when the supply of oxygen is diminished because of the lack of circulating red blood cells it is essential to keep the patient who has lost a good deal of blood cool so that the demands for oxygen are kept to the minimum. The old treatment by blankets and hot water bottles is condemned because among other changes it increased the oxygen requirements and fluid loss from sweating.

Once the blood volume has been restored the patient will warm up naturally as the vasoconstriction disappears.

Heart and lungs

Any condition affecting normal oxygenation of the blood, such as lung congestion, pneumothorax, or haemothorax, will produce hypoxia which, in the presence of a diminished blood volume and, therefore, reduced cardiac output, will increase the danger of circulatory failure.

All the First Aider can do is to maintain adequate lung ventilation by ensuring a clear air passage and assisting ventilation artificially in suitable cases.

Heart disease due to incompetent valves or coronary thrombosis reduces cardiac output, and this is made worse by blood loss.

Additional measures

Vaso-active drugs

Vasoconstrictor drugs may mask the signs of hypovolaemia and are rarely used.

In anaesthesia, however, vasodilation occurs and this may so drop the blood pressure in a hypovolaemic patient as to prove fatal unless rapid blood transfusion is given. In such cases a vasoconstrictor drug may be helpful.

Vasodilator drugs may be necessary when the central venous pressure is high, or the urinary output inadequate after the blood pressure has been restored to normal.

Steroids

These may be helpful in hypovolaemia which does not respond to restoration of the blood volume. This lack of response occurs particularly in 'septic shock' in which there is increased capillary permeability. Steroids may prevent this increased permeability but should always be given with antibiotics.

Shock

'Shock' is a term which is difficult to define for it really indicates a dynamic clinical syndrome characterized by change due to a reduction in circulatory blood volume which causes inadequate capillary circulation leading to cellular changes.

The changes of falling blood pressure, rising pulse rate, a cold clammy skin, clouding of consciousness, diminished urinary output, vomiting, unconsciousness and even death, have long been familiar. In the sixteenth century Ambroise Paré gave an accurately detailed description of this collapsed state, which he called sowning.

Degrees of shock

Mild shock is produced by a loss of 10–20 per cent of the circulating blood volume and is easily treated by restoring the volume of blood by plasma or other intravenous fluid.

Latent shock has already been mentioned and is a term used to indicate that the development of severe shock is imminent unless treatment is rapid and adequate. It may be said to be present when the circulatory volume has been diminished by 30 per cent but the patient is still relatively fit.

Severe shock is easily recognizable and usually develops after 30 per cent blood loss. Treatment of this stage is urgent because delay will result in failure to respond adequately to transfusion and is associated with intravascular coagulation resulting from a clotting defect due to consumption coagulopathy which leads to irreversible shock, which is a state which results from too little and too slow a replacement of the blood volume. For treatment to be effective the cause as well as the clinical state needs treatment and there are many causes of shock.

Causes of shock

Traumatic, oligaemic and hypovolaemic shock are terms used to denote blood or plasma loss following injury or burns.

Cardiac shock is due to the failure of the heart to act as an efficient pump. This is seen most frequently in coronary thrombosis when an area of heart muscle becomes ischaemic and fails to contract normally.

A pericardial effusion will restrict the heart volume and therefore the cardiac intake and so the cardiac output.

Toxic shock is the result of toxins or sepsis which cause high temperature and a warm skin due to vasodilation, so that the blood is pooled with diminution in the circulatory volume and reduction in the cardiac output. It is seen in septic conditions, i.e. genito-urinary infection and septic abortion or in fevers, i.e. diphtheria and tetanus.

Neurogenic shock is a psychological phenomenon brought on by emotion, experiencing pain, hearing bad news, or the sight of some disaster producing vasomotor collapse. It is seen in fainting. The only clinical difference from the shock syndrome described above is that the pulse rate is slow. Recovery occurs when the patient lies down. At one time this was called 'primary shock' because it occurred with any trauma or severe pain. It is obviously under nervous control, the vagus nerve, for it comes on immediately. The 'secondary shock' was the effect of the main condition causing the primary shock and was delayed as the effects took time to develop. These terms are not now used as they are unhelpful.

Spinal shock follows damage to the spinal cord at the higher levels in the neck or upper thorax for at these levels the sympathetic fibres in the cord are divided and vasodilation occurs, producing a warm pink patient with a low blood pressure and diminished cardiac output. It is also used to denote a recoverable paralysis following spinal cord injury.

Anaphylactic shock is an extreme form of hypersensitivity on injection of a foreign protein to which the recipient has already been sensitized. Extreme circulatory collapse occurs due to pooling of blood, such as occurs in septic shock. Adrenaline, which is a vasoconstrictor, restores normal vascular tone.

Endocrine shock is really a crisis occurring in certain diseases of the endocrine glands and is basically a failure of cell metabolism. It is seen most familiarly in Addison's disease due to the primary failure of the adrenal gland. These patients show low blood pressure and a low temperature and even unconsciousness.

Obstruction to blood flow in a large artery in the systemic circulation produces immediate ischaemic hypoxia which renders the capillary more permeable than normal and causes plasma to pass into the tissue spaces, where acid metabolites form. Until the circulation is restored these changes cannot affect the rest of the body, but when it is restored there is an outflow of plasma-like liquid through the leaky capillary wall and a consequent fall in blood volume. At the same time acid metabolites and other potentially harmful substances enter the circulation and may so aggravate the effects of oligaemia on the kidney that it fails. This sequence of events can follow ischaemia caused by severe crushing of muscle—the crush syndrome—and similar changes occur as a result of general hypoxia that develops when the heart stops.

Effects of oligaemia on other injuries

Unconsciousness can follow bleeding and can also occur from head injury; difficulty then arises in deciding whether the unconsciousness is due to bleeding or to head injury. Blood transfusions will benefit the case of blood loss but not the head injury.

Pain

The appreciation of pain is much diminished in the severely injured so that other injuries, not bleeding, may not be complained of initially and may only come to light when the blood volume has been restored to normal. For example, rupture of the bowel with quite severe peritoneal soiling may not cause any abdominal rigidity and so be missed until later.

The pulse and blood pressure

These may be conflicting, for in head injuries with increased intracranial pressure, the pulse is slow and the blood pressure is high whereas the reverse is the case in blood loss; the head injury may not appear, from these signs, to be as severe as it is. Hence the importance of not taking any signs of blood loss in isolation.

The absence of expected signs in a person suffering from haemorrhage should not exclude the possibility of a particular injury. The First Aider should not therefore underestimate any injury just because the signs are few or absent.

5

FRACTURES AND DISLOCATIONS

FRACTURES

Definition and classification

The time-honoured definition of a fracture refers only to the bones; the fact that the bones are immediately invested by periosteum and closely related to other important soft tissues is acknowledged only in the definition of open and complicated fractures. It is not going too far to say that no fracture is simply a break in the continuity of bone because there is inevitably damage to the soft tissues, even if only to the vessels and nerves within the bone and running between it and the periosteum. With some fractures, the damage to the soft parts greatly outweighs in importance the damage to the bone itself. A crack in the skull is of negligible importance compared with a haematoma or cerebral laceration beneath; a broken rib is less important than an associated haemothorax. pneumothorax or ruptured spleen, liver or kidney.

Much of the present practice in specialized fracture units is based upon a clear appreciation that the soft parts may dominate the treatment of a broken bone. First Aid books have rightly stressed the dangers of open fractures and of causing further damage by careless handling of broken bones but they have not laid enough stress on other aspects that are of great and sometimes urgent practical importance, for example, the amount of bleeding and consequent oligaemic shock that follows all but mild and single fractures. Another relevant matter is the manner in which bones are broken.

It is customary to classify fractures according to their complexity and mobility and according to whether or not there is penetration of the skin or mucous membrane. By far the most important distinction is between open and closed fractures because the risk of infection alters the whole attitude towards treatment. The terms 'simple' and 'compound' are more misleading than informative and should be abandoned.

Whether or not a fracture is of the greenstick, impacted or comminuted variety is less important in First Aid than whether the fragments move on each other. It is not suggested that this be tested, only that it is likely to become obvious during examination and treatment. Clearly movement is more serious than fixity and more specific in its needs in treatment.

The nature of the forces that break bones is not usually considered much beyond distinguishing direct from indirect violence. A clearer idea of how bones break can be gained from recognizing the simple facts that they can be bent, knocked, twisted, pulled, pushed or crushed. The pattern of fracture follows from the forces applied, and several may occur in combination.

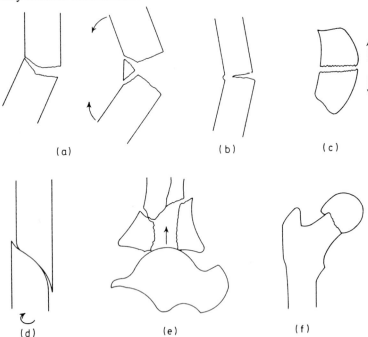

(a)   (b)   (c)

(d)   (e)   (f)

Figure 5.1. How bones are broken: (a) Bending; (b) Bending–greenstick; (c) Pulling; (d) Twisting; (e) Crushing–disruption; (f) Crushing–impaction

Bending a bone usually breaks it more or less transversely, though the line of fracture often branches once or twice (*Figure 5.1a*). A simple transverse crack right across the bone is usually caused by a sharp localized blow. Traction or avulsion fractures have a straight, transverse direction but there is a wide gap because the soft tissues are torn and the fragments are kept apart by resting muscular tone (*Figure 5.1c*). In other types of fracture muscular tone causes over-riding, not separation.

Twisting a bone makes it break along a spiral path (*Figure 5.1d*) and pushing or crushing makes it shatter or crumble (*Figure 5.1e*).

A greenstick fracture, which occurs in children, (*Figure 5.1b*) is a variant of the fracture caused by bending; an impacted fracture (*Figure 5.1f*) is a variant of the pushing variety.

Occasionally, disease weakens a bone so that it breaks more easily and even so that it gives way slowly without a distinguishable moment of fracture. The pattern of fracture varies with the state that the disease brings about but there are the same basic types as in healthy bones.

The presence of absence of important damage to nearby structures depends on the force of the injury and the displacement of bone that results.

Presented in this manner, fractures should be brought into line with everyday experience of things that break or are broken and become subjects for intelligent comprehension rather than mystical awe. Perhaps the First Aider has not been clearly taught that broken legs and fractured tibiae are the same, even though he may understand that 'a break' is not worse than 'a fracture' (or vice versa).

Symptoms and signs of fracture

The symptoms and signs that are usually taught leave no room for failing to diagnose bones that are well and truly broken, but the only invariable sign of fracture is localized tenderness over bone and even this may be masked by thick coverings of muscle and fat. This is usually accompanied by swelling with or without bruising but may be so slight as to be thought inconsistent with fracture. The signs and the pain may be thought to be owing to bruising only, or, if near a joint, to a sprain and suitable for treatment without reference to a doctor. It must be stressed, however, that this casual attitude may have dangerous effects, because some apparently trivial injuries may be serious. This applies particularly to certain fractures in the thumb and fingers, to the fractured scaphoid and to some fractures at the ankle.

When one comes to consider the effects of violence upon a bone and its surrounding structures, the range of variation of the symptoms and signs follows logically.

The anatomy of fractures

In the mildest form of fracture the bone is merely cracked and only a few vessels within it and between the bone and periosteum are torn. There is slight effusion of blood and slight stretching of sensitive structures. The bone may feel to be without abnormal movement. Even with radiographs diagnosis may not be certain for a fortnight or so, by which time an imperceptible crack will have widened or a subperiosteal reaction become evident (*Figure 5.2*).

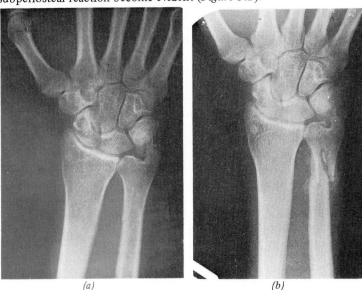

(a)   (b)

Figure 5.2. (a) The fracture may be almost imperceptible at first; (b) a few weeks later it is unmistakable

With larger forces the bone is displaced and the periosteum torn; swelling is greater and more widespread, abnormal movement and crepitus can occur and closely adjacent skin or mucous membrane may be breached. With larger forces still, local disruption and damage are increased and more distant structures and organs may be injured as well. The torn soft tissues bleed and the swelling that accompanies a recent fracture of a limb is caused by this bleeding (*Figure 5.3*). The amount of swelling can be measured and found to correspond closely with a simultaneously measured fall in blood volume. In practice, deformity of a broken limb can make swelling difficult to estimate and in the very early period after fracture little swelling will have occurred. Nevertheless, the fact that a limb is noticeably deformed means that it has been at least fairly badly injured. With fractures of the ribs, spine and pelvis, the bleeding may be great though masked by the large bulk of the region.

Complications

Bleeding and swelling

These are matters of great importance because the more serious fractures of the larger bones cause severe oligaemic shock. *Figures 4.8, 4.9* and *5.3* show swelling (and therefore internal bleeding) that is fairly typical of fractures in those regions. Bleeding is unlikely to exceed a donation or two within ½–1 hour of the infliction of the fractures shown and shock need therefore be only anticipated. With open fractures, especially if there is much damage to the soft tissues, much more severe and rapid

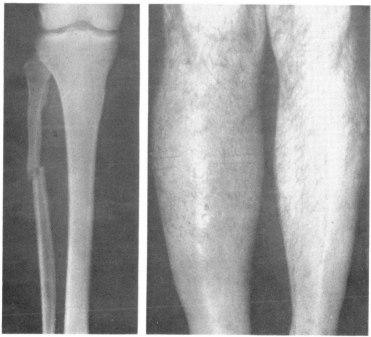

Figure 5.3. Severe swelling accompanying an otherwise unimportant fracture of the fibula; the combination of the injuring force and the tight stretching of the skin caused blistering over the fracture. This is the sort of case in which it may be advisable to clear out all the blood without delay

bleeding will occur. It must also be remembered that two or three fairly mild fractures in the same person can cause as much bleeding as one severe one. With present conditions on the roads it is not exceptional for there to be two or three major fractures as well as wounds and other injuries. It is in such cases that bleeding assumes overriding importance.

Swelling is also important because it may be so great as to stretch the skin tightly enough to stop its circulation and so kill it. This is even more likely if the skin has already been injured by crushing, abrasion or being stripped from the underlying tissues. This last can occur without fracture and results in a large subcutaneous cleft that will become distended by a large quantity of blood. A firm dressing applied early may prevent much of this bleeding and so save the skin.

Vascular damage

Swelling can also embarrass the circulation of the limb as a whole by compressing the main vessels. Pulsation should be sought in the arteries beyond the injured area. If it can be felt there is no immediate cause for anxiety but the examination should be repeated frequently and preferably by the same observer. If pulsation cannot be felt it may be because the tissues between the artery and the examining finger are too swollen to transmit the pulse.

The following signs are reassuring even though the pulse cannot be felt.

1. Warm, pink skin that blanches when pressed and promptly regains its colour when released.
2. Painless active or passive movement of joints beyond the fracture.
3. No tenderness of muscles in the injured area.

Danger signs

These are:

1. Blue skin that blanches and regains its colour slowly. White skin is even more ominous.
2. Inability to move joints beyond the fracture and great pain if passive movement is attempted. It is not necessary nor desirable to attempt any but a small range of movement and it is sufficient for movement to be tested only in the fingers and toes.
3. Hard, woody and very tender muscles in the region of the injury.

These are signs that Volkmann's ischaemic contracture is occurring. The condition is most frequent and best known in the flexor muscles of the forearm as a complication of injuries at the elbow but it can also occur in the calf as a result of fracture here or in the thigh. The cause is a reduction of the blood supply to the muscles and unless the circulation is quickly restored the muscles gradually undergo replacement by fibrous tissue, which contracts to cause severe deformity. The exact manner in which the circulation within the muscles is impeded is still argued but the signs and the dangers are beyond argument.

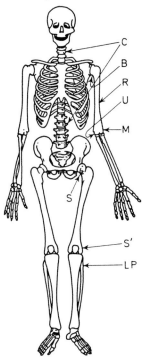

Figure 5.4. Sites of fractures and dislocations that are liable to injure nerves

C: Spinal cord and nerves
B: Brachial plexus; dislocation of the shoulder is well known to injure the circumflex nerve but the entire brachial plexus, or any part of it, may be damaged. The axillary artery may also be damaged
R: Radial nerve
U: Ulnar nerve ⎱ The brachial artery
M: Median nerve ⎰ may also be injured
S: Sciatic nerve
S': Sciatic nerve or its principal branches. The popliteal artery may also be injured
LP: Lateral popliteal nerve

Fortunately, the condition is rare and unlikely to confront the First Aider unless the patient's move to hospital is delayed. There is not much that First Aid can do to prevent or treat the condition, for which it may be necessary to expose the artery and to decompress the swollen muscles, but the following measures should be applied.

1. Try gently to correct any obvious deformity and support the limb comfortably.
2. Release any clothing or bandages that constrict the limb.

3. Expedite transfer to medical care whether these measures have helped or not. The condition may recur.

Neural damage

This should be suspected when the injured person cannot move or cannot feel properly beyond the fracture, passive movement is possible and painless, there is no pain or tenderness in the muscles and they are not hard. All feeling may be lost or there may be only patchy numbness. Paralysis and numbness may occur separately or together.

The nerves most often injured are shown in *Figure 5.4*.

As far as First Aid is concerned, there is no special treatment but it is helpful for the doctor to know roughly the extent of the paralysis and numbness when the patient was first seen.

Other complications

These include penetration of the skin and damage to internal organs that will be described under the fractures concerned. Delayed thrombosis is not likely if the patient can be moved promptly to hospital, but in other circumstances it may occur and give rise to signs already described under vascular damage. Delayed union, non-union and malunion are outside the scope of First Aid.

General principles of treatment

Being a break in the continuity of tissue, viz. bone, a fracture is rightly to be regarded as a wound and subject to the same principles of treatment as are familiar in the management of injuries in soft tissues. For these it has long been accepted that the injured structures must be brought and held together by stitches of one kind or another but it is only in recent times that the use of direct 'suture' of bones has been practised and come to be accepted as a legitimate and at times necessary method for treating fractures successfully.

'Sutures', wherever used and in whatever tissues, can fairly be regarded as splints; 'sutures' for bone include encircling loops of wire, screws, plates and nails of various kinds. Their purpose is to provide secure splintage and they can do this more effectually than any form of external splintage. This is not to suggest that external splintage is unnecessary, unsuccessful or outmoded by internal methods of fixing fractures. It is the case, however, that some fractures rarely unite without internal fixatives and that others stand a better chance of successful union and successful return of function if treated in this way.

The purposes of internal fixation are:

1. To fix fractures that cannot be immobilized by external splintage. The neck of the femur is the outstanding example.
2. To stabilize the skeleton of a limb that has suffered severe injuries of the soft tissues. It may be pointless to sew up skin, nerves or tendons in a limb that is still capable of abnormal movement. If the fracture becomes displaced stitches may tear out or grafts slip and fail to take. This applies both to immediate and to delayed repair of the soft parts. Having a rigid framework also allows movement of the limb as a whole to be started earlier than is possible with external fixation and so reduces stiffness and other disorders of function. This does not apply only to the limbs.
3. To facilitate treatment of other injuries. Fractures of the limbs that can be treated without cumbersome splints do not interfere with the necessarily active nursing of, for example, paraplegia or injuries of the chest or head.
4. To free elderly and aged people from pain and to enable them to move about and even to get out of bed within a few days. This is of great value in preventing such frequent and potentially fatal complications as pulmonary embolism, bed-sores and bronchopneumonia.
5. To accelerate recovery by rendering a limb capable of use sooner than with external splintage.

There is still a good deal of argument about the use and safety of internal fixation of fractures and the two main dangers are infection and an adverse effect upon the speed of union. These are weighty arguments and require careful consideration but it is nevertheless true that, properly used, internal fixation has been of great value in the treatment of many difficult fractures and in saving limbs and even life itself.

It can fairly be said that the wide ranges of types and severities of fractures throughout the body can nearly be matched by the wide range of methods of treatment available. In this range of methods the use of blood to combat oligaemic shock is of great importance because of the large quantities of blood that may be lost even with closed fractures and without operation.

The influence on First Aid

The increased resort to a direct surgical attack on fractures has not altered in any way the need for good First Aid but it has led to alterations in emphasis on the details of treatment.

The aims of the First Aider must be to avoid further damage; if necessary, to dress wounds and stop bleeding and to render the patient comfortable. It is also of great value if information can be given about the amount of deformity of a broken limb when it was first seen, how much bleeding had occurred and whether there was anything to suggest serious damage to the nerves or vessels of the limb. Such information may have a decisive influence upon the choice of treatment in hospital. A limb that has been very severely deformed has suffered a great deal of damage; even though the skin is apparently unharmed the circulation has sometimes suffered mortal injury and extensive gangrene may ensue.

With the possibility of operation or at least anaesthesia in mind and with the knowledge that most fractures of large bones carry the risk of oligaemic shock, careful handling and speedy transfer to hospital are of basic importance.

Handling a broken limb

This is necessary to correct severe deformity, to apply splints and to move the patient. It is little taught even among doctors but it deserves careful attention.

It is widely believed that a broken limb is intensely painful. This need not be so. The pain is most often of a dull, aching nature and by no means intolerable if the limb is at rest and not much deformed. Sudden and careless movement of the limb by the patient or an attendant causes severe pain and also causes most people to tense themselves and even writhe about, thereby increasing the pain.

The key to comfortable handling of broken limbs is relaxation by the patient and slow, deliberate actions by the attendant. Given these conditions limbs can be handled with little discomfort even though sometimes the fragments can be both felt and heard to grate on each other.

Before a broken limb is handled, the patient should be encouraged to relax and if he does he will usually agree that the limb is at once less uncomfortable. In order to achieve even this degree of success it is necessary to have the patient's undivided attention. This means that the consoling companion of a child, for example, must be asked to sit quietly by without attempting to soothe the patient or otherwise distract its attention from the First Aider.

Once relaxation has taken place the patient should be instructed to concentrate his attention on the limb and continue his efforts to relax. While these instructions are being given the attendant's hands should be laid upon a painless part. Any tensing of the patient, whether of his face, jaws or hands, should at once be pointed out and relaxation enjoined once more. Once the hands are on the limb without causing discomfort they should be moved gently so as to enable a firm grip to be established above and below the fracture. All the while the patient should be urged to relax and gently encouraged. Each step taken by the First Aider without causing the patient to tense himself or to feel

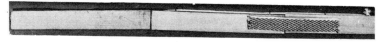

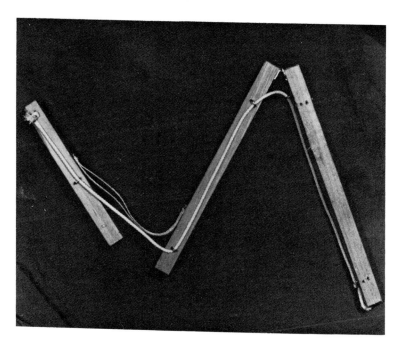

Figure 5.5. A simple device for simulating a fracture. The cord represents a neuro-vascular bundle. When this is well padded and is enclosed in the sleeve of a coat or the leg of a pair of trousers it presents the First Aider with a 'limb' that allows all deformity to be corrected but which will give way unless it is correctly handled

pain is a step towards success. The limb is moved with gentle traction applied and with the hands so disposed as to support and steady it.

If at any time the patient moves or tenses himself, the First Aider should stop and coax him into relaxing before proceeding.

First Aiders often ask if they should correct deformity. In most cases there is none worth correcting or, as with greenstick fractures, it requires considerable force. An attempt should be made to correct deformity (a) if it is very severe; (b) if the skin is tightly stretched over a bony prominence and blanched thereby; or (c) if there is evidence that the circulation is seriously impeded.

Any correction that can be carried out gently and with no more than slight discomfort is unlikely to do harm and may do a great deal of good. Correction should not be attempted if it causes much pain or if it cannot be carried out gently. In these cases deformity will have to be maintained even though the bone is protruding and other dangerous conditions are present.

The successful handling of painful limbs is something that cannot be learned except by handling broken and otherwise injured limbs. No amount of putty, plasticine or bread plastic 'deformity', or apparently protruding bone, nor any amount of acting by however skilled a casualty simulator will give the person handling a limb the feel of one that has really been injured. Some performances and some teaching aids make it only too clear that those concerned have no idea how a broken limb and its owner really behave. More effort could and should be made in pursuit of realism (*Figure 5.5*).

Splints and splintage

This has long occupied a prominent place in the practical training of First Aiders and it seems likely that it originated in the days when First Aid began and wooden splints were much used in the definitive care of fractures. The First Aider could often do almost as much as the doctor in his management of the simple fracture. With modern methods of treating fractures the gap between First Aid and definitive treatment has widened and the former emphasis on rigid splintage has been much reduced.

As far as First Aid is concerned, the purpose of splinting is to steady a limb and thereby to render the injured person comfortable and to reduce the risk of further damage by the broken bones. The combination of relative comfort and avoiding further damage helps to stay the progress of shock. If these purposes can, as is often the case, be achieved without formal splinting, none is required and this could perhaps be brought home more forcibly if the word splintage were replaced by the words comfortable support. A lower limb can be bound to its fellow but will often be best comforted and steadied by being allowed to remain where it is and packed round with pads or rolled up clothing, pillows and so on. A sling or pinning the sleeve to the coat will suffice for any fracture in the upper limb even when the patient can walk about.

Splints should not be used simply because they are available or can be improvised; this is particularly important if splinting will delay the movement of a seriously injured patient to hospital. Splints are most useful when an injured person has to be moved far or in difficult circumstances, for example, down a mountain, over rough ground or in a mine. Here again, however, it is required only for the lower limb and for the spine in as much as the patient should lie on a firm, flat surface.

Wooden splints are readily adaptable, light and easily carried. Gooch's splinting is particularly convenient because it can be wrapped round the limb, suitably padded, to give support in all directions. The Neil Robertson stretcher is essentially similar but larger and more robust and is provided for various civilian and Service rescue teams. It has had several successors that are less cumbersome and less likely to deteriorate with age but more expensive. One of the most successful as a means of providing

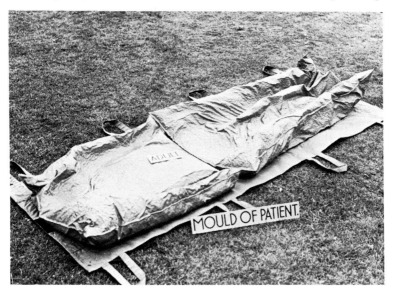

Figure 5.6. A deflatable splint after being moulded to the shape of the person lying on it

comfort and support is the vacuum mattress or deflatable splint (*Figure 5.6*).

Thomas's splint has been of very great value for the lower limb but it is awkward to carry in a rescue kit and not easy to apply in confined spaces. Its use should, however, be known and an adjustable pattern can be made to fit most lower limbs.

Thomas's splint is one of the rare appliances that has not been improved upon, in spite of numerous modifications, since its inventor Hugh Owen Thomas felt satisfied with his trials and published a description of the splint over 100 years ago. He had already tested it for some years, having discarded several earlier versions. Its value in war was strikingly demonstrated when about 1916 its introduction into British military service almost reversed the previous 80 per cent mortality from open fractures of the shaft of the femur. In World War II it emerged again as the Tobruk splint, in which limb and splint were largely encased in plaster.

It can be applied over clothing or to the bare limb and it is still much used in hospitals. Its value in First Aid lies in the fact that by a combination of supporting slings with traction it steadies the lower limb better than anything else and enables long and difficult journeys to be made with remarkably little disturbance for the casualty.

In recent years the technique of 'countour' splinting has been introduced into First Aid. It amounts to applying ready-made strips of plaster of Paris, over the clothing if necessary, moulding them accurately to the contour of the limb and binding them in place with paper bandages. The materials are available as a set encased in a plastic bag, which can also be used to hold the water, or watery solution, with which to wet the plaster strips. This method provides a reliable means of splintage in a conveniently small packet. Because the limb is surrounded by crape paper bandages any swelling occurs in safety. The principal disadvantages, that the method takes several minutes to carry out, that it needs water, and that it makes a mess of clothing, lose much of their force when splintage is required for a long or difficult journey; a packet of contour splint is much more easily carried by First Aiders than is Thomas's splint.

Newer still in the field of splintage is the plastic inflatable splint (*Figure 5.7*). This is essentially a plastic bag that can be wrapped round the limb, kept in place by a suitable fastening and then inflated. Splints of this kind have been criticized on the grounds of expense, of liability to puncture, and of liability to crack or split if folded up. Shortcomings of this kind are likely to be overcome by the invention of suitable materials. A much more serious criticism is that the pressure in the splint may be enough to stop the flow of blood in the splinted part. Extensive clinical experience with a number of different types of splint has shown that the pressure needed to splint a fracture is considerably below the pressure that has been found dangerous in laboratory experiments. If the splint is too tight a conscious patient will complain of pain and if it is too loose he will not tolerate active or passive movement of the splinted limb.

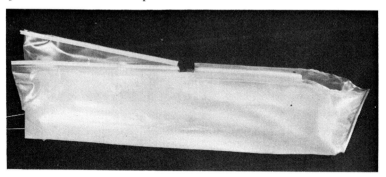

Figure 5.7. This pattern of inflatable splint is cheap and effective but the stiff closing strips make it unsuitable for folding

Inflating the splint by mouth one gets to know how hard to blow to achieve the right pressure even in an unconscious person. A pump should not be used unless the pressure within the splint can be measured. It should be between 20 and 30 mmHg. For training, pressure gauges can be used to enable the students to get to know the feel of both blowing up and palpating a splint at the right pressure. Another simple and reliable test is to raise the splint by a hand under the heel; if it buckles it is not sufficiently inflated, if it does not buckle the pressure should be reduced until buckling just occurs. This test should always be carried out if the patient is unconscious.

The ideal splint has yet to be produced but it would be cheap, transparent, tough and flexible so that it could be rolled or folded repeatedly and stored for a long time without deterioration. It should be entirely transradiant with a simple, reliable valve. It would leak above a pressure of 30 mmHg.

Inflatable splints are most useful for injuries at and below the knee and although they can be used with injuries below the elbow it is questionable whether they offer much advantage over a sling in most cases. They do not seem to be of use with fractures at other sites.

They can be applied over clothing and dressings and when applied to a deformed limb they either correct the deformity with notably little discomfort or they adapt themselves to the deformity without loss of efficacy. Inflatable splints are increasingly accepted by the medical profession and the voluntary aid societies in the light of a good deal of favourable clinical experience that has dispelled much of the criticism that the splints attracted from those that had not put them to practical use.

It is worth considering whether the word immobilize should be used as much as it is. The most that many surgeons' splints can achieve is merely to reduce the amount of movement taking place at the site of a fracture. True immobility is possible only in special circumstances that put it far beyond the reach of First Aiders, whereas the comfortable support of painful limbs is well within their powers and the use of this term might given them a clearer idea of what they are aiming at and how to set about it.

Two points of detail are worth mentioning because they conflict with accepted practice. It is stressed that an injured person must be told to lie still. It is not as a rule harmful to ask a casualty what movements he can carry out and to get him to assist the First Aiders as far as he can. Many a patient wheeled into hospital trussed on a stretcher can move himself to a couch or bed with only a little help once his bandages have been removed. For this reason, the single-handed First Aider will be well advised to make what use he can of the patient's own powers. If a lower limb has been injured it may be better not splinted or secured until the patient is on a stretcher. Firstly, once the legs are tied together the patient must be lifted bodily; and secondly, even with a full team of trained attendants it is often difficult to move the patient without causing pain in the injured limb. There need be no hesitation over detailing one person to look after the injured leg and to ensure that it moves 'in one piece' with the rest of the patient, whether he moves himself or is moved by others. This applies equally to moving a person when no stretcher is available and to cases in which both legs have been broken. A broken arm should be secured in a comfortable position on the trunk.

Comments on standard First Aid methods of treating fractures

This section deals only with fractures of the limbs. The jaw, skull, ribs, spine and pelvis will be dealt with in later chapters.

The intention is not to reject out of hand the methods laid down in present manuals of First Aid because it would be unfair to candidates for examination and participants in competitions to teach them what is not officially recognized. The general instructions regarding diagnosis and precautions are admirable but it is worth examining the standard methods of treatment against the background of what has gone before in this chapter and indicating the directions in which official policy might be changed.

The clavicle

The official method may give the impression of aiming to reduce deformity by trying to lever the lateral fragment outwards over a pad below the axilla. Even if such an effect could be achieved without obstructing the brachial artery it would have no useful effect upon the position of the fracture. The displacement is, in fact, difficult or impossible to reduce except by lying the patient down with a firm pad between the scapulae. This should be tried if sharp fragments are pressing hard upon the skin. In practice, the deformity is usually accepted and some surgeons go so far as to dispense with any form of support, encouraging active use for the whole limb right from the start. It is sufficient, therefore, to promote comfort by bracing the shoulders back and placing the arm in a sling; it does not matter whether this is narrow, large, or of the triangular (formerly St. John's arm) type.

A very rare complication of a fractured clavicle is damage to the subclavian artery. Much local swelling, with or without visible bruising, and obliteration of the pulses in the limb call urgently for medical aid.

The scapula

Fractures of this bone are usually treated by immediate active use and for First Aid a sling is as much as is needed whether the body, neck, spine or acromion process is broken.

Other fractures in the upper limb

The distinction between cases in which the elbow can and cannot be bent without causing pain is admirable. The use of bandages to secure the arm to the trunk is an unnecessary refinement. A triangular sling or pinning the sleeve with the limb in a comfortable position will meet all the needs if the patient can sit or walk. If he is lying down a sling is not usually required.

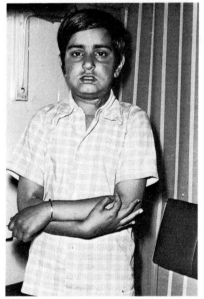

Figure 5.8. The good-arm sling

If no sling can be improvised the patient can use the other limb to support the injured one, wherever it is injured (*Figure 5.8*).

Fractures of the thigh and leg

The emphasis on arranging and supporting the injured limb as comfortably as possible is sound, but in competition work and examinations knowledge of the authorized manner of splinting is tested and many First Aid workers retain this method more prominently in their minds than the simpler one. It is still questionable whether it is more comfortable to leave the injured limb that has been splinted separate from its fellow than to bandage the two limbs together.

Fractures of the patella

The limb is most comfortable when the knee is straight but the bandage applied to cross behind and pass above and below the patella in front cannot be expected to have any useful effect on the separated fragments.

Crushed foot

There is little to be gained by splinting the foot as described in the event of there being a wound, because fractures in the foot are not usually easily moved.

DISLOCATIONS AND FRACTURE-DISLOCATIONS

Dislocations may be regarded as fractures in which displacement has occurred between two bones that are normally in contact. From this it follows that many of the signs and symptoms of fracture will be present. There is, however, often less damage to the soft tissues than with fractures, therefore less bleeding into the injured area and therefore less shock. The only serious exception to this is dislocation of the hip because in the adult great force is required to dislocate this structurally strong joint and the bulky surrounding muscles are extensively torn.

With dislocation a joint may be mechanically locked; this is usually the case with the jaw, fingers and hip. In the shoulder, elbow and ankle it is often possible for the patient to carry out a little movement. With fracture-dislocations the range of passive movement may be considerable but the patient will not willingly move the joint himself. It is not suggested that a joint that is known or suspected to have been injured in this way should be subjected to passive movement, but the point is stressed because when a limb is first examined in search of injury it may be fairly easily movable at the joints and in the unconscious or severely shocked patient there may be no reaction to show that the movement has caused pain. Also, the restless, unconscious patient may move injured joints enough to dispel suspicion.

The main signs of dislocations and fracture-dislocations are pain and swelling at a joint; neither fixity nor inability to move the joint is essential to the diagnosis. As with fractures, vessels and nerves may be damaged, but dislocations are rarely open.

The shoulder

1. Dislocation of the acromioclavicular joint follows a violent blow on the point of the shoulder and is not infrequently produced by falls on the rugby football field or in the wrestling ring. The deformity is characteristic (*Figure 5.9*). It is not produced by upward movement of the clavicle away from the

scapula but by downward and forward movement of the scapula as the weight of the arm pulls it round the curve of the chest. The patient can usually be persuaded to brace his shoulders back and will be much comforted as the deformity is almost

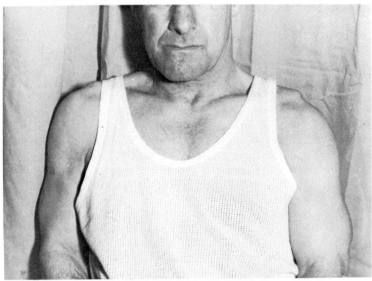

Figure 5.9. Deformity of acromioclavicular dislocation. Old dislocation on right; larger step of recent injury on left. The patient was a wrestler

completely overcome. A sling may be added to take some of the weight. The deformity and discomfort are much reduced if the patient lies on his back.

2. Occasionally the inner end of the clavicle is displaced. It usually comes forward as a hard bulge at the root of the neck. Rarely it goes backward and may press on the jugular or carotid vessels behind. Recumbency or a sling is all that is needed.

3. The scapulohumeral joint is one of the most frequently dislocated. Epileptics and sportsmen may suffer recurrent dislocation and be able to effect reduction themselves. There is no need for First Aid in such a case but the patient should be advised to see a doctor with a view to having further dislocations prevented by operation.

Except in fat people, anterior or subcoracoid dislocation is usually recognizable on sight because of the characteristic flattening and angularity of the affected shoulder. A little movement may be possible;

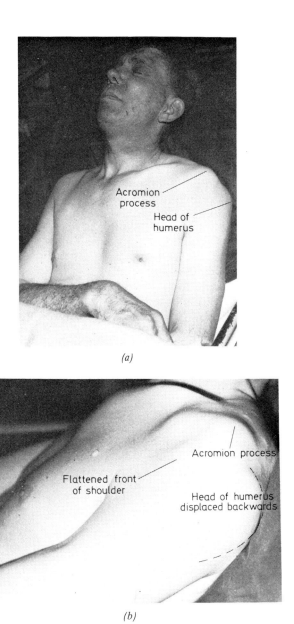

(a)

(b)

Figure 5.10 (a) (b). Posterior dislocation of the left shoulder

the presence of crepitus or much swelling suggests fracture-dislocation. The brachial plexus may be damaged and the effect varies from paralysis of the deltoid muscle to paralysis of the entire limb with all sorts and degrees of motor and sensory disturbance in between. Rarely, the axillary artery is bruised or torn, causing pallor and cyanosis of the limb, which lacks arterial pulses and gradually cools and becomes painful. Damage to nerve or vessel urgently requires treatment.

Posterior dislocation is rare and easily overlooked except in a thin person, when the shoulder is obviously deformed (*Figure 5.10*). The shoulder may be locked in medial rotation. Pain and fixity are sufficient grounds for suspecting this and any other injury of the shoulder that requires medical attention (*see* Chapter 6).

The only First Aid required is to support the arm in the most comfortable position. This may not be necessary for the spontaneously reduced recurrent dislocation but it should be provided and medical attention advised if a fresh dislocation has been reduced.

It is rightly stressed that the First Aider should not attempt to effect reduction but it can sometimes be enabled to occur if the patient lies prone with his arm hanging free over the edge of a stretcher, couch or bed. This is a safe and comfortable position and is worth using if the patient is already lying or is in much pain when in some other position.

Luxatio erecta is the rarest and most arresting type of dislocation. The shoulder is locked with the arm pointing straight upwards. One can do no more than try to make the patient comfortable.

The elbow

Most often the point of a dislocated elbow sticks out prominently behind. The forearm may also be displaced to one side or the other with the skin tightly stretched. Some movement is always possible and sometimes the joint is like a flail. The forearm is consequently supported by the sufferer. The brachial artery and median, ulnar and radial nerves may be injured. A pointing forefinger indicates median paralysis because this nerve supplies all the muscles that cause flexion of the forefinger.

The treatment is as laid down for fractures of the upper limb but lying prone with the arm supported and the forearm hanging free is comfortable, safe and may allow reduction to occur spontaneously.

The wrist

Dislocations of the wrist are rare and deformity is often masked by swelling (*Figure 5.11*). A triangular sling is all that is required of the

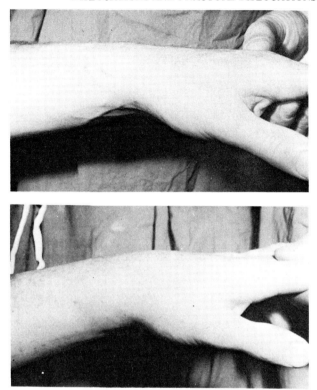

Figure 5.11. The lower photograph shows no more than slight swelling accompanying fracture-dislocation of the wrist. The normal wrist is above, the print being reversed to facilitate comparison

First Aider but an inflatable splint gives better support and may be used unless there is numbness and tingling in the hand and fingers. This means that a nerve has most likely been injured; treatment is required urgently and additional pressure may be harmful.

The digits

Dislocated digits are often locked but are sometimes put back by the patient and it may then be possible to move the digit almost normally. No First Aid is required but the patient should see a doctor because serious and disabling damage may have occurred (*see* Chapter 6).

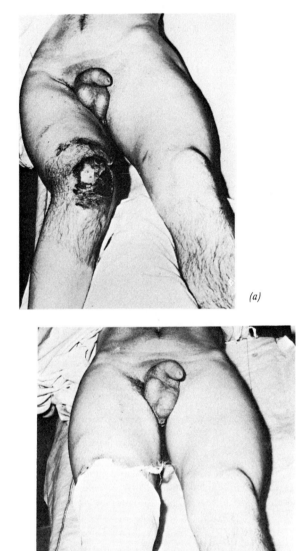

(a)

(b)

Figure 5.12. (a) Posterior dislocation of the right hip
caused by a blow on the bent knee. (b) The relationship
of the limbs to each other and to the trunk is in striking
contrast to what is shown by (a)

The hip

Dislocation is most often backwards and the limb is flexed, adducted and medially rotated at the hip so that the knee lies flexed across its fellow in the position adopted by models when posing (*Figure 5.12*). There is pain and a hard lump (the displaced greater trochanter) in the buttock.

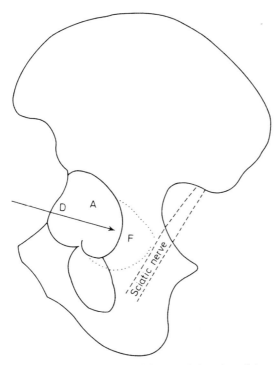

Figure 5.13. The danger of fracture-dislocation of the hip to the sciatic nerve. D: Direction of the dislocating force. F: Region of fracture at back of acetabulum (A)

Fracture-dislocations do not lock the hip and the limb may be in a natural position but appear slightly shortened. The buttock is swollen and tender. There may be numbness, tingling and weakness caused by damage to the sciatic nerve. Fracture-dislocations are increasingly frequent from road accidents in which great forces are applied along the flexed thigh of driver or passenger and drive the head of the femur through the posterior margin of the acetabulum (*Figure 5.13*).

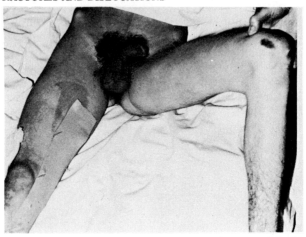

Figure 5.14. The typical posture of anterior dislocation of the hip. Note the mark of impact on the inner side of the knee

Anterior dislocation of the hip is rare but usually produces an obvious and characteristic deformity (*Figure 5.14*).

The knee

1. Genuine dislocations of the knee are rare and may gravely injure the popliteal vessels and nerves. The joint is strikingly deformed and locked. Treatment is very urgently required. Less rare are severe tears of the ligaments and capsule. There is no deformity and there may be remarkably little swelling or pain at first; the patient may even move the limb and hobble on it. Lameness following a knee injury requires medical advice; comfortable support is all the First Aid that is required. Walking is better avoided (even when it is possible).

2. Dislocation of the patella produces obvious deformity, weakness, fixity and pain. It may occur on the sports field and may be recurrent, especially in girls. Recurrent dislocation is usually easily reducible by extending the knee fully and the patient may know this and play on. Medical advice about a curative operation should be recommended.

The ankle

Simple dislocation of the ankle is extremely rare. Obvious deformity is usually caused by fracture-dislocation. The displaced foot may be locked out of place with skin tightly stretched over bone (*Figure 5.15*). Replacement can sometimes be achieved easily by gentle traction with the patient relaxed and may even take place during examination. Such joints are very wobbly and should be carefully supported in as nearly

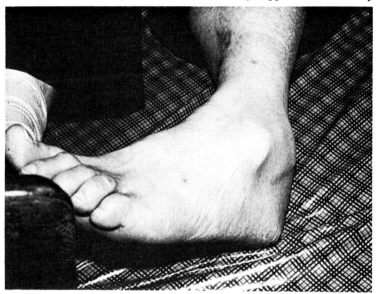

Figure 5.15. Fracture-dislocation with skin dangerously stretched

the normal position as possible. Sometimes stretched skin can be eased by lying the patient prone and allowing the foot to hang freely over a firm pad placed in front of the ankles. This position is safe and comforts the ankle; tense muscles relax and the foot may slip back into place. This should be explained to the patient lest he be taken unawares and jerk the foot out of place again.

The foot

Dislocations of the foot are rare and the deformity is usually fixed; it may be striking or masked by swelling (*Figure 5.16*). The swollen, painful foot that prevents walking requires medical attention without delay because some of these injuries can have disastrous consequences.

The role of the First Aider

Proportionately more space has been devoted to dislocations and fracture-dislocations than is allotted to them in manuals of First Aid because the pictures they present are a little more variable than is described. Nevertheless, many dislocations can be diagnosed with assurance and the typically misshapen appearances of joints can usefully be added to First Aid teaching; they should add interest without overburdening the syllabus.

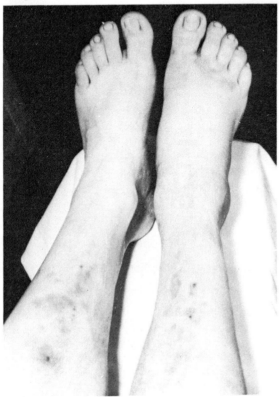

Figure 5.16. Fracture-dislocation at the middle of the right foot. The abnormal direction of the fore part of the foot and the toes is evident in spite of swelling

It is perhaps unnecessary at the simplest level to distinguish between fracture-dislocations and fractures because their obvious features are closely similar, but some fracture-dislocations have complications (for example, sciatic paralysis at the hip) that do not occur with either fracture or dislocation alone.

The unorthodox postures described for dislocations of shoulder, elbow and ankle are not widely known and play no part in present

First Aid teaching but they are comfortable and safe and may reduce deformity and pressure on skin, nerves and vessels without danger.

SUMMARY

Fractures and dislocations usually cause pain, swelling, deformity, abnormal movement and loss of power. It is not usually difficult to recognize that injury has occurred; the precise diagnosis is often irrelevant but danger signs must be *known, looked for* and *acted on* when present. They are:

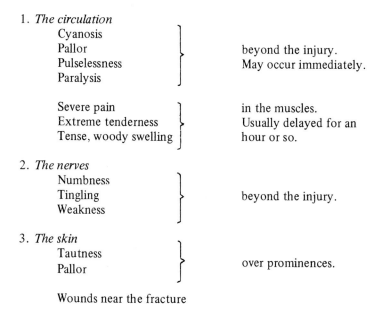

1. *The circulation*
   Cyanosis
   Pallor   beyond the injury.
   Pulselessness   May occur immediately.
   Paralysis

   Severe pain   in the muscles.
   Extreme tenderness   Usually delayed for an
   Tense, woody swelling   hour or so.

2. *The nerves*
   Numbness
   Tingling   beyond the injury.
   Weakness

3. *The skin*
   Tautness
   Pallor   over prominences.

   Wounds near the fracture

Fixed deformity should be comfortably supported. Splints other than inflatable ones are usually not applicable; a sling may suffice or the patient may be better off lying down.

Movable deformity can often be corrected with advantage provided that the hands are used carefully, the patient's co-operation is gained and pain is avoided.

A cautious attempt to correct deformity may be made if it is movable and the danger signs are present. This advice is perhaps better restricted to those who are frequently dealing with injured people rather than for the keen amateur to whom a suspected fracture is a great event except in a competition or an examination.

Formal splintage is rarely necessary but because it must be known it tends to be invested with excessive importance. The textbooks' admirably judicious attitude towards it requires careful emphasis and the understandable tendency of the eager to display their prowess may need to be restrained.

It is not always necessary or desirable to forbid movement. What the patient can do without discomfort is unlikely to do harm and may be a valuable guide to the First Aider.

A single severe fracture or several milder ones can cause serious bleeding either internally or through an associated wound. The signs of shock may come on quickly at any time after injury.

Many fractures require treatment under anaesthesia. For this and the preceding reasons the patient should be sent to hospital without delay and without being given anything to eat or drink.

6

MINOR INJURIES

GENERAL CONSIDERATIONS

Minor injuries can be regarded as those that have a tendency to spontaneous recovery with little or no treatment. The difficulty lies in deciding correctly that an injury is unimportant. A wound, for example, may appear small but penetrate deeply, opening into joints or the trunk or it may divide nerves or tendons of the hand. Its situation is important: a stab wound of the abdomen may produce a small and apparently superficial wound in the abdominal wall whereas in fact the point of the instrument has gone far enough to pierce the bowel. Soiling of the peritoneal cavity ensues, but if it appears that the wound has not penetrated the full thickness of the abdominal wall suspicions may not be aroused until serious complications have set in.

Injuries of the small joints of the digits may appear trivial if they produce few signs, whereas they may have far-reaching effects if important ligaments have been ruptured. Then they will result in instability of the joint under stress, as in rupture of the collateral ligaments of the metacarpophalangeal joint of the thumb. Such an injury inadequately treated may result in permanent weakness of grip and seriously handicap a manual worker.

Serious injury may occur in larger joints such as the cervical spine, but apart from pain and stiffness there may be few physical signs so the condition is regarded as a sprain whereas in fact a dislocation of the cervical spine may be present (*Figure 6.1*).

A further source of error in diagnosis occurs in patients with multiple injuries. Often no complaint is made of less painful injuries and so certain areas may not be examined. Such errors in diagnosis can be avoided only by careful history-taking, full examination and an appreciation of the anatomical structures that could be affected. In these cases, however, responsibility for diagnosis falls wholly on doctors and not on First Aiders.

The diagnosis of a minor wound may be correct, but incorrect treatment may lead to serious complications so making a minor wound

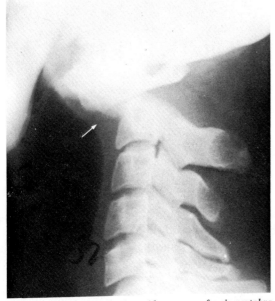

Figure 6.1. Fracture of odontoid process of axis vertebra. Displacement to this extent occurred after a dive into shallow water. For several weeks the victim complained only of a stiff neck

a major problem. This is seen in small wounds of the fingers leading to tendon and joint infections. Similarly some minor closed injuries may be more adequately treated by operation if the full significance of the apparently trivial is appreciated.

Repair

All wounds whether closed or open heal by fibrosis or scar tissue. The aim in treatment should be to minimize the amount of scarring by close approximation of the divided structures, because scarring is unsightly on the skin and may seriously interfere with function if deep and situated near a joint. The delicately balanced and co-ordinated movements of the fingers may be lost if scar tissue is formed from a relatively small wound in relation to the interphalangeal joints; accurate repair by suture will minimize this and restore good function.

Infection must be avoided by early, thorough toilet and surgical cleansing of a wound, because infection increases the tissue destruction and therefore increases the amount of scar. The wound and, more important, the skin around it, are thoroughly washed under aseptic conditions with soap and water and to prevent further contamination the wound should be closed. In most cases this can be achieved by simple suturing or by the use of sterile, adhesive strips of microporous material. If there is loss of skin, skin grafting is necessary, because the skin is the best barrier to infection.

For the most part the wounds are open or closed according to the integrity of the skin. Sometimes, however, the skin has been so injured that its blood supply has been permanently damaged and it will die. This allows infection to occur. Such wounds are regarded as potentially infected even though at first sight they have intact skin cover (*Figure 6.2*). As soon as the dead skin becomes demarcated from the healthy skin, it should be excised together with any underlying dead tissue and the area grafted with a split skin graft.

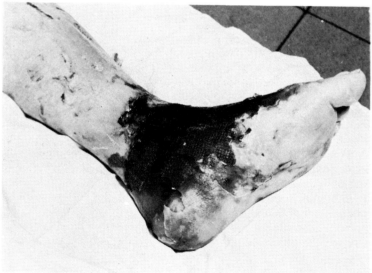

Figure 6.2. Closed injury of the foot, followed by skin necrosis

The important consequences of minor wounds are fibrosis and infection. These should be minimized as far as possible.

The fear of infection in turning a closed wound into an open one by an act of surgical repair is likely to lead to second rate results owing to fibrosis. With full aseptic precautions the risk of infection is less serious than the poor results from failure of adequate repair.

The fear of infection in open wounds frequently leads to inadequate treatment when, in fact, early, thorough cleansing and removal of dead and foreign material diminishes considerably the risk of infection.

The temptation for First Aiders to poke and pry into wounds to remove foreign matter in an attempt to avoid hospital treatment cannot be too strongly condemned, because it increases the likelihood of infection and may add more bacteria to those already present.

Briefly then:

(*a*) small open wounds should never have more than simple washing and a dressing from First Aiders.

(*b*) if there is any doubt whatever about the depth of the wound it should only be dressed and seen as soon as possible by a doctor. This applies most of all to wounds of the trunk, hands and those lying near joints.

Bruises

Most bruises are trivial and require no special treatment other than, possibly, a firm bandage. Bruising results from extravasation of blood into or beneath the skin following injury and some bruises are so large and extensive that they accommodate 10 or even 20 per cent of the total blood volume (*Figure 6.3*). Bruising is frequently seen where bone lies directly under the skin, as in fractures of the ankle, the hip, the elbow and the upper end of the humerus; these bruises are always associated with much more pain than would be expected from a bruise alone and this should raise suspicion of a fracture and require more careful examination and possibly a radiograph.

Still more important are certain bruises of the soft parts of the abdominal wall that occur because the abdominal wall has been driven hard against the pelvis or the posterior abdominal wall. Such bruising takes on the pattern of the garment next to the skin and can be compared with the pattern stamped onto a medal or coin. It is important because for the skin to have been so bruised the abdominal contents may have been caught and injured between the abdominal wall and the bony 'anvil' of the spine or pelvis. Laparotomy is usually indicated by this sign alone.

Bruising may appear in the groin within an hour or so of injury such as fracture of the pelvis. Sometimes larger vessels are ruptured so that more blood is extravasated into the damaged tissue; this collects in the damaged area and forms a swelling, the pressure of which stops the bleeding. Such swellings are called haematomas, and they differ from bruises only in degree. Frequently they are situated deep in the tissues and do not cause discoloration of the skin. The blood clots and forms a firm swelling; later this liquefies and forms a fluid swelling which is then slowly absorbed, possibly taking 4—6 weeks to resolve completely.

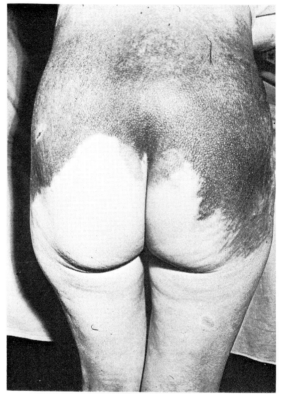

Figure 6.3. A bruise this big may remove a third or more of the blood in circulation

If the haematoma is in close relation to a bone it may undergo calcification, form a hard swelling and feel like a bony tumour. This takes several weeks to develop. The reason for the calcification is difficult to determine; it is thought to be associated with damage to the bone or periosteum and this is supported by the fact that all calcified haematomas are closely related to bone. It is in a sense ossification though the bone so formed usually differs microscopically from normal bone structure and resembles callus round a fracture.

Haematomas close to the bone are more painful than in the soft tissues because of the pressure they produce on the periosteum covering the bone. Similar pain can arise with local swelling from infection of the bone, a condition known as osteomyelitis, which may come to light after an apparently trivial injury. A useful diagnostic characteristic is that if pain occurs immediately after the injury it is likely to be caused by bruising whereas if it is not felt until several hours later it may be the first sign of osteomyelitis. The diagnosis, therefore, of a haematoma is not always easy and such cases should be referred to a doctor for opinion, particularly if the pain seems to be out of proportion to the degree of violence, or if it increases after a day or two. Local warmth occurs with haematoma or infection; so does tenderness, but it is much greater with infection than with haematoma.

A bruise must not, therefore, be too lightly dismissed by the First Aider for it may overlie a more important injury. Haematomas may require aspiration or incision for evacuation if the tension on the skin is too great.

Foreign bodies

In wounds

The variety of foreign bodies that have been found in the tissues is remarkable. They are most easily removed shortly after entry because the track of the larger foreign bodies can usually be followed without difficulty. The size of the wound is no guide to the size of the foreign body because this depends on the size, the shape, the velocity of the penetrating foreign body and the elasticity of the skin. The First Aider must not, therefore, be misled and assume that because the wound is small the foreign body is small.

Whenever a foreign body has or is thought to have penetrated the skin, the patient should be referred to hospital for X-ray examination. Its direction and depth cannot be determined by examination of the wound. In most cases the foreign body is removed surgically under full aseptic precautions, particularly if it is lying in relation to important structures. If, however, a relatively small foreign body has penetrated deeply into muscle, it can often be regarded as harmless and left alone. It could be removed surgically but most likely after an extensive operation which may cause more damage to the tissues than the foreign body is ever likely to cause; even the most apparently obvious foreign body can prove to be unexpectedly elusive and the decision whether to seek it or leave it must be made by a doctor.

Failure to remove a foreign body may result in a sinus forming; that is, the wound does not heal but continues to discharge pus owing to local infection carried into the tissues by the foreign body. One of the most persistent causes of a sinus is clothing being carried into the tissues by the foreign body, because clothing is usually heavily infected and is not opaque on radiography. In time the foreign body may be expressed and the wound heal, but more frequently it requires surgical removal by opening up the track formed by the sinus.

In natural orifices

Children are notorious for pushing foreign bodies into their noses or ears or putting them in the mouth and swallowing them.

The nose

The judicious use of pepper is often a simple remedy for foreign bodies in the nose.

Foreign bodies should be removed by a doctor, because there is a real danger that the inexperienced person may push the object higher up the nose causing it to be impacted, or may push it backwards into the nasopharynx. From here it could easily be inhaled, causing obstruction of a bronchus, or at a later date an abscess if it is not removed.

The ear

Any foreign material in the ear will cause infection and ulceration; for this reason it must be removed. Removal of foreign bodies is difficult, requiring special lighting and instruments, and if care is not taken the drum can be permanently destroyed. Therefore the First Aider should never attempt to remove anything from the ear.

The mouth

Swallowed foreign bodies are commonplace and there seems to be no limit to the variety of objects which reach the stomach (*Figure 6.4*). For the most part foreign bodies which reach the stomach will pass naturally. The difficult part of the passage is down the oesophagus and round the curve of the duodenum. If a patient states that he has

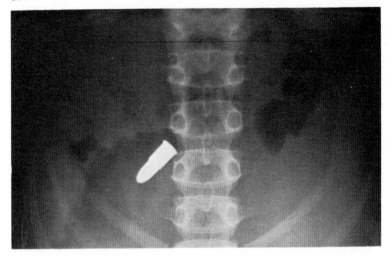

Figure 6.4. Radiograph showing a live 0.38 bullet in boy's stomach

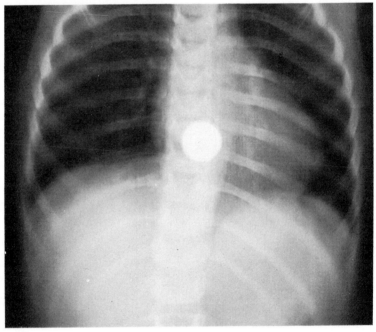

Figure 6.5. Radiograph showing an old halfpenny (2.5 cm in diameter) in the oesophagus

swallowed some unusual foreign material, he must be sent to hospital for an X-ray examination. If the foreign body has been arrested in the oesophagus (*Figure 6.5*) then it can and must be removed; this is done with a special tubular instrument with a light on the end down which forceps can be passed to remove the offending object. Small dentures, if swallowed, nearly always become arrested in the oesophagus owing to their jagged shape, and many dentures are made of plastic which is not radio-opaque. The patient is rightly insistent that he knows where the object has stuck and points to the correct level. This is an important sign that a foreign body is present but, if as has occurred, dentures become displaced during sleep the patient may awake complaining of a sore throat, with no thought of having swallowed a foreign body.

If the object negotiates the oesophagus the next danger point is the duodenum for this is narrow and curved and it is in negotiating the curves that the object may stick. The Kirby grip is commonly seen on X-ray examination; being nearly straight, it is most likely to stick in the duodenum of very young children and requires removal, because if left it may perforate the sharply curved bowel, with serious consequences. Knowing the risk, it is justifiable in many small children to remove the Kirby grip from the stomach before it reaches the duodenum; hence the importance of having these patients sent to hospital early.

The decision whether a swallowed foreign body requires removal or not depends on its shape, size, consistency and possibly on its toxicity.

In adults most foreign bodies that get as far as the stomach will pass naturally and are better left alone and observed on X-ray film at regular intervals. Only if one becomes arrested should operation be considered. Sometimes very large foreign bodies do reach the stomach and warrant removal. It is surprising how large an object can pass down the oesophagus; for instance, a 6-inch Biro pen has been removed from the stomach of a child aged 2½ years. It seemed inconceivable that it could have been swallowed and it was certainly impossible for so large an object to negotiate the duodenum. It was difficult to credit the history but fortunately parts of the pen were visible on X-ray film (*Figure 6.6*).

Some swallowed foreign bodies such as small coins, beads, marbles and so forth are harmless, but open safety pins, pins and needles are a potential source of danger and better kept under observation in hospital because they may perforate the intestine and give rise to peritonitis. Small, smooth objects can be ignored if swallowed. No special diet is necessary or effective for swallowed foreign bodies and medicines should be avoided.

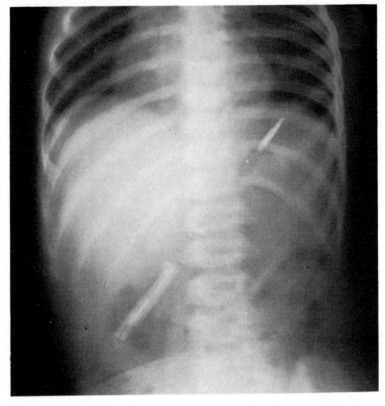

Figure 6.6. Radiograph showing a Biro pen in the stomach of a child aged 2½ years

It is often the chest rather than the abdomen that should be radiographed in search of a foreign body.

Inhaled foreign bodies

Inhaled foreign bodies must be removed because they give rise to lung abscess and obstruction or ulceration of the trachea or bronchus. The commonest object to enter the trachea is a small denture, perhaps carrying one or two teeth only. Other small objects may be inhaled and are associated with varying signs from choking, coughing, wheezing and stertor to cyanosis and even asphyxia, depending on their shape and size. An X-ray examination in such cases is essential; some apparently 'swallowed' foreign bodies are, in fact, inhaled and the presence of any of the above symptoms is an important point in the diagnosis. Most foreign bodies fortunately are opaque to X-rays and are therefore easily diagnosed and can be removed. Some objects, especially small plastic dentures are not seen with X-rays. These cases must be treated according to the history and if the patient is in no doubt about having inhaled something or complains of retrosternal pain or any of the above symptoms bronchoscopy must be performed for diagnosis and removal if any object is seen. Vegetable matter is often particularly dangerous.

The urethra and anus

The objects that have been found in the bladder are of great variety and too numerous to list. They are usually passed into the urethra for erotic

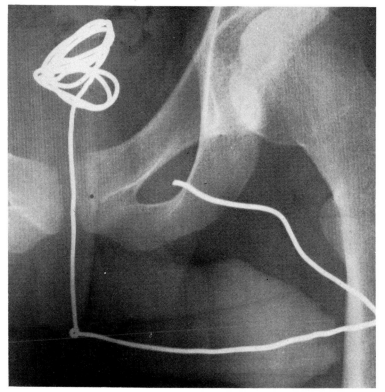

Figure 6.7. Radiograph showing soft 'solder' wire in bladder and urethra

stimulation and either slip out of the grasp and enter the bladder or cannot be pulled out and so are pushed in for fear of discovery. If the foreign body is still presenting at the urethral orifice, no attempt should be made to remove it, for if it were removable the patient would have done this himself and much damage may result to the urethra from trying forceful extraction (*Figure 6.7*). Strapping can be used to prevent any presenting object from disappearing. These patients and those who have a history of inserting some foreign material into the bladder should be sent to hospital at once for full examination with radiographs and possibly cystoscopy. Most of these objects can be removed only by opening the bladder. They must be removed before bladder infection because this may eventually go on to kidney infection and cause serious illness.

Foreign bodies in the rectum are not infrequent and a great variety have been described. No attempt should be made to remove them by the First Aider because it is a painful procedure and not without danger of perforating the rectum, which is a most serious and often fatal injury.

MINOR OPEN WOUNDS

As in all open wounds, the risk is infection. When the wound is large the seriousness of the condition is appreciated more readily and consequently more care is taken. Minor open wounds, on the other hand, tend to be neglected.

The first point to establish in a small wound is that the wound is minor and that no arteries, nerves, joints, tendons or body cavities have been entered. If the First Aider can satisfy himself on these points, though often he cannot, then definitive treatment for the minor wound can be undertaken. This should consist of thorough cleansing of the wound and surrounding skin with soap and water and the application of sterile dressings. The dressing should be kept dry until the wound is healed because a moist dressing allows bacteria to penetrate the wound. So far no adequate porous waterproof dressing has been devised. The usual difficulty in minor wounds of the hands is that the dressing may easily become moist from work or toilet. Moist dressings should be changed at once, but the less frequently they need changing the better, for each change may allow bacterial contamination. Impermeable dressings should not be used for more than an hour or so, because they prevent evaporation and so make the wound moist.

A small cut on a finger may allow bacteria to enter and form a small abscess which may extend to involve the tendon sheath. This may result in a serious general condition, ending in a crippled hand. Deaths from tetanus number over 100 a year in this country and many of the wounds from which tetanus results are so trivial that they are neglected; tetanus rarely follows the larger wounds because they receive prompt and skilled attention.

Tetanus prophylaxis

The problem of preventing tetanus is a difficult one, but prophylaxis must always be borne in mind with any open wound (*see* page 44).

MINOR CLOSED INJURIES

It is often difficult to differentiate between strains, sprains, ruptured ligaments, minor fractures and other allied painful conditions near joints. In the lay mind the term 'sprain' is applied to any painful condition near a joint which does not look like a fracture. There is danger in this because there may have been a minor fracture or torn ligament which require rather more energetic treatment than a sprain.

More dangerous still, however, is the fact that infection of bone may be brought to light by a minor injury and treated as a sprain. To the more wary, however, the degree of pain from bone infection is out of proportion to the severity of the injury and the onset of the pain may be delayed for 12 or more hours after the injury.

It is as well, therefore, to define the terms and deal with them on a regional basis.

A strain

A strain is really no more than the stretching of a normal ligament or muscle beyond its accustomed range, but without tearing any of its fibres, so that no swelling is associated with a strain.

A sprain

A sprain goes a stage further and is associated with tearing of some of the fibres of ligaments, muscles or joint capsules, but not complete rupture. These injuries are associated with local swelling and tenderness over the point of injury. Bruising may appear later and distal to the injury.

Rupture of a ligament

Rupture of a ligament means complete loss of continuity of a definite anatomical ligament and, correctly, the particular ligament should be named. Where a ligament has been ruptured the joint concerned is usually unstable and can be completely or partially dislocated depending on the joint involved. A ruptured ligament is therefore associated with local pain, tenderness, swelling and joint instability, though the instability may be masked by muscle control or muscle spasm for a while.

A dislocation

A dislocation is usually accompanied by rupture of one or more ligaments and tearing of the joint capsule when the joint goes out of place. It may stay there or slip back so that the true nature of the injury may be missed.

A minor fracture

A minor fracture may produce one or more of the above signs; that is, pain, tenderness local swelling and possibly deformity. A minor fracture may be small in size but of great importance. Does the fracture matter? Will it influence treatment? A small flake of bone pulled off by a ligament is correctly a fracture, but treatment is for the torn ligament, not the flake of bone. Conversely, a fracture may easily be dismissed as a bruise or sprain, when in fact the fracture is important. A fracture of the scaphoid may well simulate a sprain and be diagnosed only when, several weeks later, the painful wrist is no better. This is an important small fracture which requires correct treatment initially and may even then give rise to prolonged disability. The rather confusing group of signs and symptoms may be clarified if it is recognized that with all these 'minor' injuries they arise mainly because soft tissues are torn whether there is a fracture or not. Deciding which injuries are important is something that the First Aider will be well advised to leave to a doctor.

THE UPPER LIMB

The shoulder

Clavicle

Fractures are common and usually easily diagnosed because the bone is subcutaneous and the local pain and tenderness and deformity are obvious. Difficulty may, however, be experienced in the young with a greenstick fracture because the bone is still in continuity and may therefore only present local pain and tenderness. This is true of all greenstick fractures, so children require especial care in assessment of their injury (*see* treatment on page 103).

Dislocations

These may occur at the outer end of the clavicle, where the clavicle forms a joint with the acromion. Dislocation at this joint produces a lump at the outer end of the clavicle, because the scapula loses its normal fixation to the clavicle and drops to a lower level (*see Figure 5.9*, Chapter 5). This injury should be treated by the application of a sling to support the arm and the patient sent to hospital; operative repair may be necessary in severe cases.

Injuries of the rotator cuff

Four muscles, the subscapularis, the supraspinatus, the infraspinatus and teres minor arise from the scapula and pass laterally, being inserted into the head of the humerus, which they cover as a tendinous hood

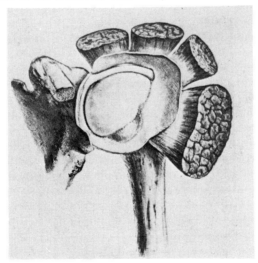

Figure 6.8. Formation of the rotator cuff (seen from inside the joint)

(*Figure 6.8*). Their individual actions produce varying degrees of rotation of the humerus; together they initiate and assist the deltoid muscle in abduction. Rupture of one or more of these tendons causes weakness or loss of the power of abduction. Rupture results from injury when the cuff is degenerate. Degeneration progresses as age advances and is marked after the fifth decade. The degree of trauma necessary to cause rupture depends on the degree of degeneration. At the age of 40–50 years quite severe force is required to produce a cuff tear. Sudden jars or wrenches such as occur in falling or trying to preserve one's balance are often responsible. In extreme old age the rupture may result from simple elevation of the limb.

The main symptoms are pain and weakness of the shoulder. There is no deformity and the condition is frequently dismissed as a sprain, and the arm rested in a sling. In actual fact the rupture of the cuff is a serious injury because it causes prolonged disability and pain. If the shoulder is treated by rest stiffness is added to these symptoms and increases greatly the problem of restoring shoulder function. Treatment should be conservative and active but operation may be indicated. So, for the First Aider, a shoulder which has weakness of abduction or pain after injury requires attention in hospital, whether the injury is severe or trivial. Other conditions may simulate a cuff tear but cannot be diagnosed without suitable X-ray examination.

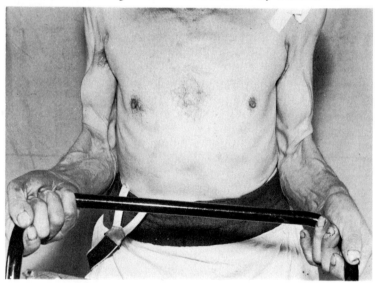

Figure 6.9. Bilateral rupture of the long heads of the biceps

The arm

Rupture of the tendon of the long head of the biceps muscle occurs in the elderly, in whom the degenerate tendon easily gives way. The rupture causes loss of attachment of part of the biceps muscle so that contraction of the muscle results in the belly of the muscle contracting into a firm and obvious swelling in the lower part of the arm, which is larger and lower than normal (*Figure 6.9*). The pain is felt over the upper third of the arm and is followed by bruising that tracks downwards. There is not usually much pain or weakness and it is frequently dismissed as a bruise or a strain. Treatment, as in most degenerative conditions, is generally graduated active use and re-education, but operation is sometimes indicated.

Rupture of the lower end of biceps is much less frequent but because the whole of the muscle is put out of action (with rupture of the long head the muscle is still partly effective) it is best treated by operation.

The elbow

The elbow is a hinge type of joint and subject to many and varied injuries as a result of blows and falls on the elbow or outstretched hand.

Gross injuries, like dislocations and displaced fractures, are clinically obvious.

The lesser injuries of sprains, ruptured ligaments, traumatic synovitis and minor fractures are often difficult to differentiate clinically. Some of these minor fractures are of considerable importance because they may interfere with function if not properly treated initially. If the elbow has a full range of movements, full rotation of the forearm and is stable on adduction and abduction, then there is probably no significant lesion. If the joint is unstable then there may be an avulsion of the medial or lateral epicondyle or a ruptured medial or lateral ligament; the ultimate diagnosis must be by X-ray examination. If the elbow movements are incomplete there may be a fracture, small in size, which is blocking the movement and may require operative treatment. The medial epicondyle may be avulsed or the medial ligament ruptured, which allows the elbow to abduct beyond its normal range so that the head of the radius strikes the humerus and fractures. This results in pain, tenderness, bruising and instability on the medial side of the joint with a fracture of the radial head on the lateral side (*Figure 6.10*). The fracture may be missed as the pain and bruising are on the opposite side. Swelling round the joint is a sign of an important injury to it.

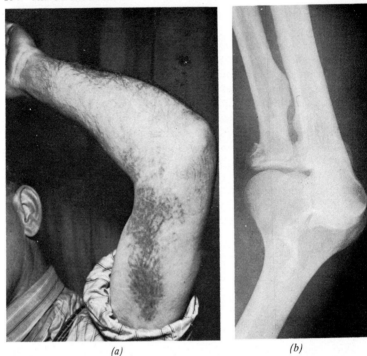

(a)   *(b)*

Figure 6.10. (a) Bruising, swelling and tenderness over inner side of elbow. (b) Radiograph of the same elbow showing fracture of the head of the radius on the lateral side. This is printed upside down so as to correspond approximately with the position shown in (a)

It is obvious from this that most elbow injuries require full examination by a doctor, as early as possible, for the exact diagnosis requires experience and almost certainly an X-ray examination.

'Tennis elbow'

This is a painful condition affecting the outer side of the elbow just distal to the lateral epicondyle. The exact cause of the condition is disputed but it results from repeated strains of the origin of the extensors of the wrist and fingers from the lateral epicondyle and capsule of the elbow joint. Housewives are affected as often as men because of the strain to which they subject this muscle group in wringing out clothes. In men, repeated use of such instruments as screwdrivers tends to produce the same lesion, as do blows and falls on the hand; tennis is rarely responsible. It is a partial tear of the muscle origin followed by fibrosis. The pain is fairly constant but aggravated by gripping and any of the actions that accompany it. The condition is not serious and in time resolves itself but this may take 18 months to 2 years. Treatment is unsatisfactory in many cases and may necessitate change of occupation temporarily. The pain associated with full elbow function, lack of bruising and swelling is usually sufficient to exclude any more serious lesion. For the First Aider, however, the signs too closely resemble more serious injury for 'tennis elbow' to be a safe diagnosis.

The forearm

Tenosynovitis of the forearm is the result of mechanical irritation of the tendons about 3 inches above the wrist. It affects the radial carpal extensors where they pass beneath the thumb extensors. It is a further example of pain following repetitive movements and is common in industry. It is not a serious condition, though painful and frequently associated with local swelling. In its early stages it is frequently characterized by a leathery creaking which can be felt when the wrist is flexed and extended. It resolves with rest, preferably by splinting the wrist. Alternatively, deep massage may be beneficial but this does not allow painless use of the arm until the condition is cured, whereas splintage allows the use of the arm without pain though the wrist is held rigid. Recurrence is uncommon.

Other painful conditions of the forearm are usually due to bony injury, either undisplaced fractures or greenstick fractures.

The wrist

Pain in the wrist following a fall is common and may be the result of a sprain, a torn ligament or a fracture. If there is no bony deformity to be felt the diagnosis can only be established by an X-ray examination. It is important that the diagnosis be established early so that proper treatment can be started. Some of the fractures are serious, notably fractures of the scaphoid. Others are unimportant though painful, notably avulsion fractures of the styloid process of the ulna, and avulsion flake fracture of the triquetral. These are injuries in which ligaments have been torn from the bone and have taken a flake of bone with them. The treatment is rest until the ligament has healed. Frequently the fracture does not unite by bone but forms a strong fibrous union which is adequate for normal function. It is difficult, however, to exclude any significant wrist injury correctly without an X-ray examination; these patients, therefore, should be sent to hospital.

Another noteworthy condition of the wrist that may be characterized by the onset of pain after a wrench or jar is thickening of the sheath of tendons near the thumb and known as de Quervain's condition. There is a small, tender lump on the side of the wrist and the thumb cannot be bent fully because of pain. It is cured by a small operation.

Ganglion

A ganglion is a gelatinous cystic swelling that may be so tense as to feel like bone. The condition occurs most frequently on the back of the wrist, though it may arise in other situations, such as the ankle and foot. The swelling may be unsightly, but it merely causes aching rather than sharp pain. It follows a previous injury in which some part of the capsule of the small joints of the wrist have been torn, so allowing escape of synovial fluid. If there is pain from a ganglion it is probably due mainly to this capsular rupture, not to the swelling. It is of little importance and frequently disappears spontaneously, or it may be dispersed by sufficient pressure to rupture the cyst. Operation is rarely indicated. The commonest mistake is for these swellings to be diagnosed as a displaced carpal bone, but the fact that wrist movements are full and the onset gradual should exclude this.

The hand

The hand as a whole must be regarded as a strong, complicated mechanism of great dexterity. Injuries, even minor ones to any part of the mechanism, may result in permanent incapacity and ill advised treatment may only increase the incapacity.

Any inclination the First Aider may have to carry out definitive treatment in hand and particularly finger injuries should be discouraged. The small injury may be considered minor in importance but it may end in a major disability. Expert advice should always be obtained as soon as possible.

Injuries to the hand are common and are most important when they affect the thumb or the fingers. The metacarpal bones are easily felt under the skin, so that any major displacement of a fracture is easily seen and felt. These fractures require medical treatment and X-ray examination. Lesser fractures may show alteration in the normal knuckle outline when the fist is clenched, or swelling but no deformity or displacement; they can be treated as a bruise with a firm supporting bandage for comfort and protection, leaving the wrist and fingers free for normal active use.

The fingers

The important injuries are sprains, torn ligaments, ruptured or avulsed tendons and fractures and they are often indistinguishable from each other by the First Aider.

Sprains

These affect the interphalangeal joints and cause swelling, pain and some loss of function but no instability of the joints. No special treatment is necessary though the joint will remain swollen and uncomfortable for a considerable time.

Torn ligaments affecting the interphalangeal joints have instability added to the above symptoms, but instability is usually recognized only by skilled testing. All swollen and painful finger joints should be seen by a doctor.

Flexor tendon avulsion

Avulsion of the flexor tendon from the terminal phalanx results from muscular violence usually in a degenerate tendon. There follows inability to flex the terminal joint actively, though passively there is a full range. Early operative repair by reattaching the tendon is the only treatment likely to restore normal function.

Mallet fingers

Avulsion of the extensor tendon from the terminal phalanx results in a 'dropped finger' or mallet finger. Little or no active extension of the terminal joint is possible though the tip of the finger can be pushed up.

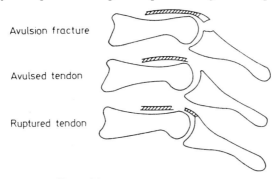

Avulsion fracture

Avulsed tendon

Ruptured tendon

Figure 6.11. Varieties of mallet finger

Treatment aims to keep the finger fully extended so that the tendon can reattach itself. The results, however, are disappointing and frequently only partial recovery occurs. Fortunately, however, this causes very little disability in the function of the hand. In some instances the tendon, as in other sites, pulls a piece of bone off the terminal phalanx (*Figure 6.11*). This deformity is unsightly and often interferes with the dexterity of the hand, so that operation may be necessary to improve the appearance and function of the finger.

Middle slip tears

More proximally in the finger the extensor tendon divides into three strands, one on each side of the middle joint and one passing over the joint and inserted into the middle phalanx; it extends the finger at

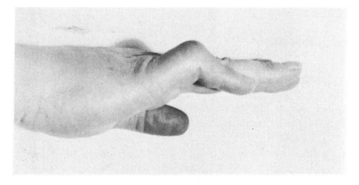

Figure 6.12 (a). Appearance of finger with a middle slip tear

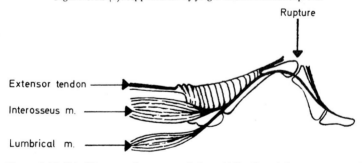

Figure 6.12 (b). Diagram of rupture of the middle slip of the extensor tendon with retraction of the torn part towards the base of the finger and with displacement of the lateral bands, which normally cross the back of the joint, towards its sides

this joint. Rupture of this tendon to the middle phalanx results in a flexion deformity of the middle joint even when the knuckle and terminal joints are held fully extended, a position no normal finger can adopt (*Figure 6.12a* and *b*). These injuries require early surgery for repair. Late repair gives poor results in comparison.

Fractures

Phalangeal fractures are important, because injury to the closely related tendons results in a stiff finger. Too long immobilization of the finger may likewise result in permanent stiffness. No matter how small a fracture is suspected, it requires early and expert assessment and treatment. There is often a good deal of swelling and this may mask considerable deformity.

It is unwise, therefore, for any First Aider to attempt definitive treatment in finger injuries because they may lead to permanent incapacity.

The thumb

The common injuries to the thumb are rupture of the inner collateral ligament of the metacarpophalangeal joint and fractures of the base of the first metacarpal.

Ruptured ligament on the index finger side of the thumb causes instability of the joint and the instability is such that the normal finger—thumb pincer grip is weakened as the thumb moves away on pressure. This injury is far too often diagnosed as a strain or a sprain. It is, in fact, a serious injury and requires expert advice. Operation may be required for the repair of the ligament. Once again, the painful swollen joint is not to be dismissed by the First Aider as 'just a sprain' to be treated by bandaging (*Figure 6.13*).

Fractures of the base of the first metacarpal are only really important if associated with deformity or, as more frequently happens, with a dislocation, although recovery can occur with conservative treatment the span of the hand may be lessened, which in a musician could be a serious disability. In a manual worker the disability might be insignificant. Such injuries require an X-ray examination and careful assessment and treatment.

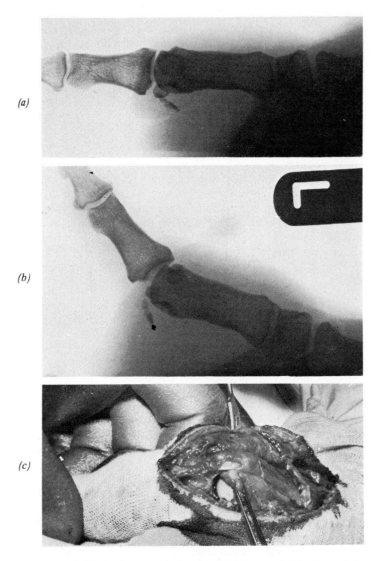

(a)

(b)

(c)

Figure 6.13. (a) Radiograph showing flake fracture of the base of the proximal phalanx. (b) Radiograph of the same thumb with abduction strain applied to the distal part of the thumb. (c) The tear in the capsule shown at operation is where the collateral ligament has been avulsed with a small piece of bone from the proximal phalanx

THE LOWER LIMB

The hip

The hip may be strained or sprained, but because it is deeply situated and therefore more difficult to examine adequately the diagnosis of strain or sprain is dangerous.

In the young there are many conditions, such as Perthes' disease and slipped femoral epiphysis, which give rise to pain and a limp, but with ability to walk and move the hip fairly freely. These are serious conditions and may require 2 years or more hospital treatment. They can be and aften are dismissed as sprains, because the child or parent will always remember a recent fall and blame this for the pain. In older people, fractures, infection and tumours may present with only pain and a limp and be called sprains. All hip conditions associated with pain require an X-ray examination whether there has been a recent injury or not.

The thigh

The thigh is subject to many blows which produce painful conditions from bruising through muscle rupture to fractures of the femur. The fractured femur is usually obvious because any movement of the leg is painful. Bruising and muscle rupture do not tend to cause severe pain on passive movement of the leg, though it may be severe if active movement is attempted. Swelling is associated with these injuries and there is local tenderness. If the muscles are completely ruptured active extension of the knee is impossible; with incomplete rupture and with bruising it is possible though painful.

Muscular violence, such as sudden extension of the leg against resistance, may cause rupture of the quadriceps in the lower third of the thigh. This occurs in the older patient, or the young with rheumatoid arthritis, in which condition there are degenerative changes in the quadriceps expansion. The condition may be virtually painless, but there is complete inability to raise the leg with the knee straight. The thigh muscles can be felt to contract and seen to form a bulge some way above the knee. Any patient who is unable to raise the extended leg off the couch should be regarded as having a serious injury some-where between the hip and the ankle, and therefore in need of hospital treatment.

The knee joint

The knee joint is so superficial and so subject to injury that a great variety of lesions can occur—sprains, ruptured ligaments, 'minor' fractures of major importance as well as major fractures and cartilage injuries. The First Aider should therefore send all knee injuries to hospital for expert opinion and X-ray examination.

Cartilage injuries are common in footballers and in certain occupations, especially those that involve a lot of kneeling, such as mining. When the cartilage tears it frequently locks the knee in slight flexion; swelling of the knee joint with its characteristic bulge above the patella ensues later. This is a very painful condition and any manipulation makes the pain more excruciating. The First Aider should make the knee as comfortable as possible—usually resting semi-flexed over a pillow is adequate—and send the patient to hospital. Any attempt to unlock the knee should be undertaken only by a doctor.

The leg

Bruising of the leg is common and may be associated with considerable swelling. Sometimes, if over bone, the swelling may be due to an undisplaced fracture, so care is necessary before deciding that only a bruise is present. If the bone is painless on trying to strain it with the hands then probably no fracture is present.

Direct injury over the upper half of the anterolateral compartment of the leg may produce a very firm swelling with pain and tenderness. This is usually due to a tense haematoma forming in an inelastic space bounded by bone and fascia. The tension can be such that the muscles in the compartment have their blood supply partly obstructed. If this is not relieved the muscles gradually die and become replaced by fibrous tissue. There is severe pain at rest and it is further aggravated by any movement of the foot or toes (*see* Chapter 5). The condition can be relieved by incision when the tense muscle will belly out of the wound, after which the skin cannot be closed because of the tension, so the defect must be covered by a skin graft. Such cases should therefore be sent to hospital for treatment (*Figure 6.14*). Mild cases, however, respond to rest, usually in a plaster cast.

Ruptured tendo Achillis

Rupture of the tendo Achillis is frequently referred to as a rupture of the plantaris tendon but in fact this tendon rarely ruptures.

The condition is dramatic in onset and the patient feels as if someone had kicked or struck the lower part of the back of the leg with a stick. He often looks round angrily to see who was responsible and perhaps is surprised to see nobody. After the accident he is only able

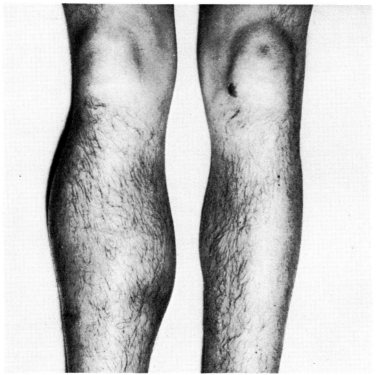

Figure 6.14. Swelling of lateral aspect of right leg

to hobble as he has no ability to 'take off' from his foot for the main plantar flexor for this action is the tendo Achillis. Nevertheless, it is not unusual for the true nature of the occurrence to go unrecognized.

In the elderly the tendon may rupture while walking. The rupture is more a pulling apart of the tendinous fibres than a clean rupture so that the tendon may feel in continuity within its sheath; hence the diagnosis of ruptured plantaris, which cannot normally be felt.

In younger persons a similar condition may develop from renewal of some violent unaccustomed sport, such as tennis at the beginning of the season. In these cases the rupture occurs at the musculotendinous junction and is a violent avulsion of the tendon from the muscle.

Much bruising and pain are associated with it at this age whereas in the elderly pain is present but rarely bruising because the tendon is degenerate and avascular.

Treatment is generally conservative; that is, the foot is supported by firm bandaging from the toes to the knee and the foot kept in a plantar flexed position by raising the heel of the shoe 2.5 cm (1 inch), or alternatively placing the leg with the foot plantar flexed in a plaster cast until the tendon has healed, which takes approximately 6 weeks.

Operation is occasionally performed so medical advice should be obtained soon but not necessarily urgently.

The ankle

Gross injuries round the ankle joint are easy to recognize by the swelling, deformity and pain. The difficulty arises in differentiating between sprains and minor fractures. Severe sprains or torn ligaments can be very painful and simulate a fractured ankle. Conversely, a fractured ankle may easily be diagnosed as a sprain. X-ray examination is probably the only method of making a positive diagnosis, but if the patient with an ankle injury and little swelling can walk, even though with a limp and some discomfort, the chances are he has not a serious ankle fracture. The exact diagnosis is often not important because it will not affect the treatment, which should consist of firm support of the ankle by bandaging to control swelling and assist weight-bearing, but it is obviously not the responsibility of the First Aider to take such a decision.

If the injury is such that the patient cannot bear weight on his foot then X-ray examination is essential because there may well be an important fracture even though it may be small and not causing any palpable deformity. Alternatively, severe ligamentous and capsular tearing may cause severe pain and inability to bear weight. These injuries are really partial dislocations which have reduced themselves, so the radiographic appearance may be normal, all the injury being in the soft tissues. This may be considerable and require operative repair. For the First Aider, however, a firm supporting bandage for all ankle injuries and a medical opinion is the best course of action.

The foot

Fractures of the toes are such frequent injuries in certain occupations that some firms supply at reduced cost steel-capped boots for protection. For the most part, however, fractures of the toes may be treated as bruises if the skin is not broken; they all heal well and cause little disability after the initial pain. The best type of splint is, in fact, a hard-soled and roomy boot which both protects and splints the toes very well. If the toe is wrapped up in bandages or plaster, wearing a boot is impossible and the patient may be rendered, by his treatment, incapable of the work that he would otherwise have continued to do. A haematoma under the nail may cause a good deal of pain and this can be relieved by piercing the nail with a heated pinpoint, so allowing the blood to exude and relieving the tension which is the cause of pain.

If the skin is broken the wound requires the usual cleansing and dressing, which may necessitate keeping the foot off the ground and hence the use of crutches.

Fractures of the metatarsals cause local pain and tenderness but heal well if weight-bearing is avoided. The exception to this is a fracture of the base of the fifth metatarsal; this may be caused by direct violence or a twist of the foot, when the base is avulsed from the metatarsal. Because of the pull of the ligaments these fractures heal slowly and frequently, like avulsion fractures elsewhere, by fibrous tissue only. In the case of a weight-bearing bone, this can cause fairly prolonged disability. The condition may closely resemble some sprains of the ankle.

Other serious injuries of the foot cause inability to bear weight and therefore require further investigation at hospital.

Stress fractures

Fractures can occur without any recognizable single cause and follow repeated minor trauma due to excess stress on the particular bone. This is seen most commonly in the second metatarsal, particularly where this bone is longer than the first metatarsal. It was of frequent occurrence in the Army and became known as a 'march fracture'. It develops insidiously with pain and local swelling over the affected area. Its true nature is only revealed by X-rays, when a fracture line is seen with early callus forming round it. It heals quickly and well if the foot is rested in a plaster cast.

A similar condition can occur in the upper third of the tibia and has been found in male ballet dancers. Footballers may develop such fractures in the fibula and many have been found in the necks of young femora. Old persons occasionally show 'stress' fractures just above the ankle. The pathology and treatment are the same wherever the condition occurs.

Stress fractures can also occur in diseased bone, particularly if the bone is curved by the nature of the disease as in Paget's disease.

The onset of pain in a bone, therefore, particularly in the lower limb, may be due to a fracture even if its onset is insidious and there is no history of any recognizable injury in the past.

FIRST AID

From the above it will be seen that the responsibility of the First Aider is to recognize that an apparently minor injury may be of major importance. It is therefore, only right and proper that he should send many simple injuries to a doctor so as not to overlook the occasional severe one (*see* Chapter 11).

Minor wounds require dressing and protection from infection; minor closed injuries require firm support either with Elastoplast or wool and firm crape bandage, but doubt as to the significance of the injury should often arise in the mind of the First Aider.

7

BURNS AND SCALDS

The outstanding effects of burns are upon the skin and the circulation, from which spring directly, complex and manifold changes throughout the organism and, indirectly, the consequences of infection.

A burn injures more or less of the skin and unless very mild it effects a breach and so comes within the definition of a wound. The wound is unusual in that while it rarely goes deep it may affect a very large part of the surface of the body and so damage a great deal of tissue, which is disposed of only slowly by natural processes and unless removed surgically invites and promotes infection. There is also loss of liquid (*see* page 153) from the circulation.

Originally applied to lesions caused by dry heat, the term burn is now used to cover many injuries inflicted on the skin by physical and chemical agents. Mechanical forces are excluded except for the friction burn, in which the obvious damage is done by the heat generated by high-speed friction that may not be sufficiently forceful to injure the skin mechanically. More forceful friction abrades without burning, but it nevertheless partly destroys the skin and causes the swelling, exudation and liability to infection and scarring that characterize the true burn.

The effects of dry and moist heat are so similar that distinction between burns and scalds will not be made. Other causes of burning such as chemicals, electricity and ionization radiations have special features.

THE GENERAL AND LOCAL EFFECTS OF THERMAL BURNS

The skin

The manner of burning

The effects on the skin depend upon the temperature of the burning agent and the duration of contact with it. Very high temperatures may merely singe and redden if very briefly applied, but will char deeply if contact is prolonged. Another important influence is the state of the circulation in the skin. Normally the skin helps to regulate the temperature of the body by allowing more or less of the blood to lose heat to the environment, but the circulation in the skin also has the ability to dissipate heat applied to the surface of the body. If there is sluggish circulation any applied heat will accumulate locally because the tissues are poor conductors; indeed, it is the poor conductivity of the subcutaneous fat that makes it a good insulator. A degree of warmth that is tolerable or even pleasant upon normal skin with a good circulation may seriously damage ischaemic skin. Herein lies the most serious objection to the use of hot-water bottles in the 'treatment' of shock and the use of layers of blanket or other wrapping offers no safeguard

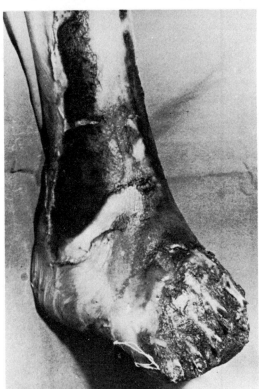

Figure 7.1. The original burn occurred while dozing by the fire. These burns are often deep and aggravated by poor circulation in elderly people

because they confine the heat and reduce the rate of cooling of the hot body; this heat slowly permeates the wrappings and may bring the surface of the skin to much the same temperature as the source of heat. In some instances the heat has penetrated deeply and it has been recorded that the liver has been cooked on its surface by a not very hot hot-water bottle applied, with the conventional 'precautions', to the flank of a profoundly shocked person.

The danger is particularly great with the old and the unconscious. The rise in temperature is so slow that it is tolerated until the pain nerve endings become injured and no longer capable of giving warning. Serious burns can occur in bed or while dozing in front of a properly guarded fire (*Figure 7.1*).

Local effects

The mildest response to thermal injury is transient vasoconstriction followed by vasodilation, which causes the erythema of a so-called first degree burn. From dilatation may spring increased permeability of the vessels, exudation and swelling. Within the skin this causes first swelling and then blisters ('second degree' burns). When the skin is merely swollen the hair follicles are accentuated as distinctly visible pits so that the appearance resembles that of pig or orange skin. At this stage of damage the burn will heal rapidly and completely in about 7 days, but if burning continues the surface appearances may not at first change perceptibly even though the damage done to the skin will have

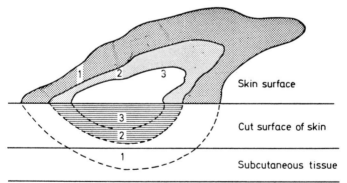

Figure 7.2. Partial-thickness skin loss, showing the three zones of damage. Zone 1 is affected by hyperaemia. Zone 2 also looks red but the circulation has ceased. Zone 3 is area of coagulation. Zones 2 and 3 will die but they do not penetrate below the skin and healing can be expected

become sufficient to destroy it more or less completely (*Figure 7.2*). With the high temperatures of flames and molten metal the skin may be killed so quickly that vasodilation and exudation cannot occur, the tissues are coagulated and vary in appearance from the dry, brown and deeply fissured surface familiar on a well-cooked joint to a hard, whitish, sunken area. With the lower temperatures of some hot liquids there is time for blistering to occur before the skin is killed. It usually assumes a mottled reddish colour.

This appearance of mottled red skin occurs because the vessels were dilated and well filled with blood at the moment of their death. Unlike the erythema of a mild burn, this redness is not affected by pressure. Sometimes, however, skin that blanches and regains its colour is in fact dead. The local circulation has come to a halt but the blood is still fluid and capable of being moved within the vessels. Later the red cells stop moving in the capillaries and the red colour is uninfluenced by pressure (*Figure 7.3*).

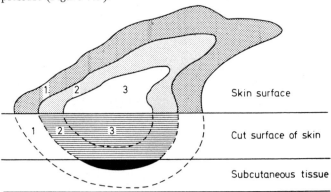

Figure 7.3. The same surface is presented as in Figure 7.2 but zones 2 and 3 extend into the subcutaneous tissue. Here, skin is totally destroyed and grafting will be required

From this description it will be evident that the surface of the skin presents appearances that may be seriously misleading. Dupuytren's description of six degrees of burning was based on appearances and the three degrees later accepted simply describe three intensities of burning of the skin's surface without regard to the depth of skin destroyed. They are of no practical value.

Recognizing the depth of a burn

In practice it is important to decide whether the burns are those that kill the skin completely or those that leave it capable of healing without scarring. In the deep group healing will occur, but the process is slow and accompanied by much scarring which is caused partly by the destructive effects of the burn itself and partly by the aggravating effect of infection that follows (*Figure 7.4*). For these burns skin grafting is required in order to achieve healing with the least risk of infection and the least amount of disfigurement and crippling by scar.

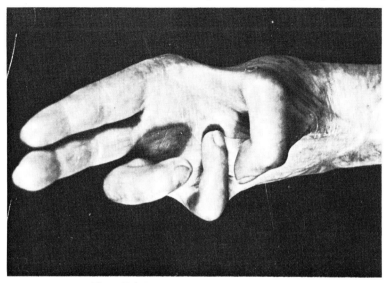

Figure 7.4. Severe contracture of the hand

Superficial burns do not need grafting because enough epithelial elements survive in the germinal layer, the hair follicles and sweat ducts, to regenerate a new surface within 2 or 3 weeks. Infection can occur and though it is not usually such a serious complication as with deep burns it can destroy scanty epithelial survivors and render a superficial burn deep.

The term superficial is used here in place of the more precise if less elegant description, partial-skin loss, and deep in place of whole-skin loss.

From what is now known about the effects of burning upon the skin it is clear that a more reliable method of determining the depth of a burn than mere inspection is desirable. The simplest is by pricking the burnt area firmly with a sterile pin. If the sensation is painful the burn will heal without need for grafting but in some parts of the body the converse it not true, so that not all anaesthetic skin has been killed by the burn. Another method is to inject a dye into the circulation

TABLE 7.1

Grid of Approximate Mortality Probabilities for Various Combinations of Age and Area

% Body area burned	Age (years)																
	0–4	5–9	10–14	15–19	20–24	25–29	30–34	35–39	40–44	45–49	50–54	55–59	60–64	65–69	70–74	75–79	80–84
78 or more	1	1	1	1	1	1	1	1	1	1	1	1	1	1	1	1	1
73–77	.9	.9	.9	.9	.9	1	1	1	1	1	1	1	1	1	1	1	1
68–72	.9	.9	.9	.9	.9	.9	.9	1	1	1	1	1	1	1	1	1	1
63–67	.8	.8	.8	.8	.8	.8	.8	.9	1	1	1	1	1	1	1	1	1
58–62	.7	.7	.7	.7	.8	.8	.8	.8	.9	1	1	1	1	1	1	1	1
53–57	.6	.6	.6	.6	.6	.7	.7	.7	.8	.9	1	1	1	1	1	1	1
48–52	.5	.5	.5	.5	.5	.6	.6	.6	.7	.8	.9	1	1	1	1	1	1
43–47	.4	.4	.4	.4	.4	.5	.5	.5	.6	.7	.8	.9	1	1	1	1	1
38–42	.3	.3	.3	.3	.3	.4	.4	.4	.5	.6	.7	.8	.9	1	1	1	1
33–37	.2	.2	.2	.2	.2	.3	.3	.3	.4	.5	.6	.7	.8	.9	1	1	1
28–32	.1	.1	.1	.1	.1	.2	.2	.2	.3	.4	.5	.6	.8	.9	1	1	1
23–27	.1	.1	.1	.1	.1	.1	.2	.2	.3	.4	.6	.8	.9	.9	1	1	1
18–22	0	0	0	0	0	.1	.1	.1	.1	.2	.3	.4	.6	.8	.9	1	1
13–17	0	0	0	0	0	0	0	0	.1	.1	.2	.3	.4	.6	.7	.8	.9
8–12	0	0	0	0	0	0	0	0	0	0	0	.1	.2	.4	.5	.6	.7
3–7	0	0	0	0	0	0	0	0	0	0	0	0	.1	.2	.3	.4	.5
0–2	0	0	0	0	0	0	0	0	0	0	0	0	0	.1	.1	.2	.3

The figures represent the likelihood of survival after burns of varying sizes occurring at various ages.
0 means every expectation of survival.
1 means every expectation of death.
Children and young adults can be expected to survive burns of 18–22 per cent, whereas old people may die from burns affecting as little as 10 per cent of the body.

to see how much of the burn does not become stained. It is obvious that these tests are not suitable for First Aiders but the following can be said of visual assessment. If there is any swelling or blistering the First Aider must regard the burn as being serious and if he should see a burn very soon after it has been inflicted, though there may then be no more than erythema, swelling and blistering can soon follow.

Shock

Local causes

The shock (other than mere fainting) that follows burning is caused in the early stages by a fall in the volume of blood in circulation. The swelling and blistering that take place in the burned area are caused by exudation from the capillaries of a liquid closely resembling plasma. The greater the mass of burnt tissue the greater the loss of liquid by exudation. Up to a point the body can compensate for a fall in the volume of circulating blood and the associated changes. The best warning that shock will be serious enough to require careful and skilled treatment is the area that has been burned. In practice, it is usual to ignore mere erythema when calculating the area of a burn but because First Aiders often see burns before blisters have had time to form this distinction should not be pressed upon them.

Children become shocked more readily after burning than do adults, but if adequately treated their ability to survive severe burns is greater (Table 7.1). If more than 10 per cent of the surface of a child or more than 15 per cent of the surface of an adult has been burned shock will be severe enough to require treatment without delay.

Estimating the size of a burn

The area of burnt skin can be calculated in two ways. For small areas, it is convenient to use the area of the patient's outstretched palm and fingers. This is 1 per cent of the total area of the body, but the area of the whole hand, palm, back and between the fingers, is 2.5 per cent of that of the body. For larger areas the 'rule of nines' is useful. In adults the limbs and trunk each have an area that is 9 per cent of the total or a multiple of 9.

The head and neck	9 per cent
The upper limbs (9 per cent each; hand 2.5 per cent)	18 per cent

The lower limbs: (twice 9 per cent each; thighs 9 per
    cent; legs 6.5 per cent; feet 2.5 per cent)   36 per cent
The trunk: (twice 9 per cent front and back)   36 per cent
                                                    ————
                                                 99 per cent

The genitals provide the remaining 1 per cent.

In children the head and neck provide a larger proportion of the surface area (up to 20 per cent at birth) and the legs correspondingly less (Table 7.2).

TABLE 7.2
Percentage Areas of Different Parts of the Body at Different Ages

Surface area	Age: 0	1	5	10	15	Adult
Head	19	17	13	11	9	7
One thigh	5½	6½	8	8½	9	9½
One leg	5	5	5½	6	6½	7

Roughly speaking, a child will require urgent treatment for shock if it has had, say, an entire upper limb burned, or half a lower limb, or a quarter of the trunk. With an adult, the dangerous area is roughly half as big again.

The clinical picture of shock

At first there may seem to be little the matter apart from the burn. Even severely burnt children sometimes arrive in hospital, crying lustily or moving about actively. Pallor may be obscured by smoke or the effects of burning but the discerning eye can usually recognize on the one hand a characteristic anxious mien and behaviour or, on the other, an ominous tranquillity.

Pain after burning is often stated to be very severe, but this is true only of superficial burns. Deep burns damage the pain nerve endings and may be painless. The misconception is most likely explicable by the fact that most people have not been severely burned; their experience has been of small burns, which can be intensely painful, and from this it has been assumed that much more severe burns must be much more painful. The victim of a severe burn is often much distressed, though not by pain. Restlessness is common, but is not necessarily caused by pain.

The treatment of shock

Essentially, this is a matter of making good the liquid lost from the circulation, usually by intravenous infusion.

These are the general and local effects of thermal burns. Burning by other agents has special effects.

THE GENERAL TREATMENT OF BURNS

The two dangers in thermal burns are shock and infection. The special dangers of other kinds of burns will be described later.

The treatment of shock

The loss of liquid from the circulation has to be made good. It cannot be stopped by any local application, whether of a 'tan' or of pressure but it gradually diminishes over the course of 2 or 3 days. Much of the liquid lost is plasma or something very similar that has seeped out of the vessels in and near the burnt area. It is now clearly established, however, that there is in addition loss of whole blood by destruction in the burnt tissues and in the circulation. Swelling begins at once and may progress very rapidly, especially in the areas where the skin and subcutaneous tissues are unusually lax and vascular (*Figure 7.5*). At first only the burnt area swells but later on the whole body may become bloated although only part has been burned.

The enormous outflow of liquid from the circulation can be matched only by comparable quantities of similar liquid given directly or indirectly back to the circulation.

The recommendation that drinking be allowed is unobjectionable if the burn is extensive enough to cause shock and if small quantities are given at short intervals. Children may have a raging thirst and if given the chance will gulp down large quantities and then vomit. Intake should be 60–90 ml (2–3 oz) an hour for children. Although the definitive treatment of shock may include salt and sodium bicarbonate solution to drink, this is not necessary as First Aid; if a drink is to be allowed it is enough that it is palatable.

The seepage amounts to roughly 1–1.5 litre for every 10 per cent of the body's surface that has been burned but the exact amount depends on a number of factors, of which age is one of the most important. Children lose larger quantities than adults for a given area burnt. The

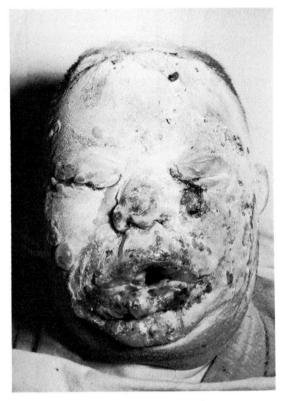

Figure 7.5(a). Early swelling after a burn of the face

rate at which liquid escapes is greatest at first and then begins to fall so that the loss during the first 8 hours is about the same as during the next 16.

The treatment of shock caused by burns is an elaborate procedure that requires close attention, repeated measurements and frequent calculations in order to restore the blood to its normal concentration and volume as quickly as possible and then to keep it normal in these respects. It will be appreciated that First Aiders cannot expect to be able to treat shock caused by burning but they should have some idea of what shock entails and of the great urgency in serious cases. Profound oligaemia and haemoconcentration can so reduce the circulation to the kidneys as to impair and even destroy their function completely.

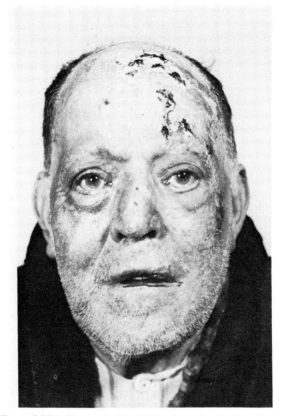

*Figure 7.5(b). Five weeks later. Note that only a little crusting
remained and the burns were fairly superficial*

Some idea of the chances of saving life can be gained from Table
7.1.

The treatment of infection

The first step in the treatment of infection is to cover the burnt area
with a clean, or preferably a sterile dressing. It is popularly believed
that air should at once be excluded and this belief is soundly based in
that at the same time airborne germs will be kept out. It must be
stressed, however, that it is not necessary completely to prevent any
contact between the air and the burnt surface. The belief that air is
harmful has promoted the undesirable practice of applying various

medicaments, often greasy, to a burnt surface. Another erroneous belief is that locally applied medication can promote healing and prevent scarring. This popular error has been lent support by misleading advertisements but there is no evidence in its favour. On the contrary, careless treatment of this kind may promote infection (*see* Chapter 3) which may in turn destroy epithelial remnants from which spontaneous healing without scar could otherwise have taken place.

Leaving burnt or adherent clothing in place avoids adding infection and leaving blisters intact maintains an epithelial barrier between the potential wound and the patient's own bacterial population on the skin. In the case of burns caused by tar and other adherent substances, firmly adherent matter should in most cases be left in place and a dressing applied over it.

If it is desirable that tar be removed—for example to unblock the nose and mouth—Swarfega is very useful.

Burns are sometimes accompanied by fractures, as when an explosion occurs or a road accident is complicated by fire. These injuries in combination should be treated each in the appropriate manner.

Once the patient reaches hospital all covering is removed and blisters may be opened. The decision is then taken about the best method of reducing the risk of infection. This decision will take account of the depth of the burn, assessing the likelihood that it will heal soundly within 2 or 3 weeks, the site and size of the burn, the degree of shock and sometimes the presence of other injuries or coexisting disease.

The choice lies between early excision of the burnt tissues, followed by skin-grafting, and the use of dressings or other local treatment. Broadly speaking, excision and grafting are carried out as primary measures when the skin has been completely destroyed over an area usually of less than about 5 per cent of the body's surface in a patient who is fit for operation. Otherwise, treatment is expectant.

Recently, it has been recommended that the best First Aid for a burn is to plunge it into or flood it with cold water because there is evidence that this may reduce the severity of the burn. It is something that can be recommended for small burns when cold water is readily available, but otherwise it is best to cover the burnt part with plain, dry dressing. Any effect that cold water may have towards reducing damage by cooling the tissues is fairly quickly lost but there is no doubt about the comfort of cooling the burned part in water and this is sufficient reason for allowing this method of treatment when it does not interfere with anything else that needs to be done. Polyurethane plastic foam has been used as a First Aid dressing for the larger burns but it does not seem to have any advantage over a clean dry sheet or cloth and would be much less readily available in most places.

Expectant treatment

Until recently it has been the practice either to cover the burnt area with an occlusive dressing (the closed method) or to leave it exposed to dry and form a crust (the open method). Both these methods have been carried out without there being any infection but this has been the exception rather than the rule. New developments include nursing the patient in filtered air that is pumped through a plastic 'isolator' tent and the use of compresses kept moist with 0.5 per cent silver nitrate solution. Maintaining a burnt person in midair by suitably arranged jets of air eliminates some of the difficulties of nursing a severely burnt person but does nothing to reduce the risk of infection.

Whichever method is used in hospital, the burnt area is first thoroughly cleansed and freed from loose skin, the remains of clothing and other foreign matter. An anaesthetic may be given for this purpose but is usually unnecessary.

First Aid is not, however, concerned with open or closed treatment; it should be restricted to covering the burnt area, apart from the face. The mask-dressing is harmless but as the face at least will be treated by exposure any dressing is superfluous. In this area, swelling is marked (*Figure 7.5a*) and will soon close the eyes. If the eyes themselves are undamaged the patient should be reassured that he will be able to see again. If the lids are not already closed over burnt eyes, small compresses moistened in tap water should be applied by the First Aider; the doctor should put in homatropine and penicillin cream.

Skin-grafting

When all layers of skin have been destroyed skin-grafting is required unless the area is very small. A small burn may be allowed to heal spontaneously because the patient will not be seriously incapacitated by requiring dressings for a few weeks and should infection occur it would not be serious. Rarely, the skin around the burnt area is lax enough to allow the burn to be cut out and the defect closed by sutures.

The treatment of contractures

The healing of skin-grafts is accompanied by the formation of scar tissue. Prompt healing, such as follows successful immediate excision and grafting of the burnt area, causes least scarring but if healing is

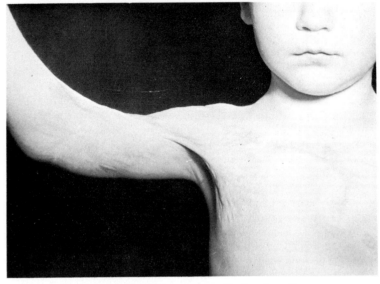

Figure 7.6. Mild contracture affecting the axilla

delayed, especially by infection, the amount of scarring will be greater. Many scars will eventually become supple and may match the appearance of the surrounding normal skin remarkably well, but where they cross joints or lie on pliable surfaces such as the face and neck they are liable to cause ugly and crippling contractures. Eyelids are pulled down, the mouth constricted, the chin drawn towards the chest, the arms and legs tethered by tight scars in the armpits and groins and the hands deformed by the pull of shrinking scars on their joints (*Figures 7.4* and *7.6*)

These scars require operation either to let in new skin or to replace them entirely by skin that will not contract. The treatment may thus extend over a matter of years and include much patient physiotherapy and training to restore function to parts that have been rendered stiff, distorted and insensitive by scarring.

The mental effects of severe burns

With such a long and painful disturbance of a person's life, schooling, work and recreation there may be considerable changes in the personality and attitude to life. These are most obvious in children, who are suddenly wrenched from their customary activities and environment to undergo a prolonged and painful and terrifying process of injections, dressings and operations in strange surroundings and without the emotional support of their home and family. No matter how sympathetic and reassuring First Aiders and medical and nursing staff may be, they cannot hope to prevent completely the emotional disturbances that result from burning and its treatment.

NON-THERMAL BURNS

Electrical burns

General effects

The victim of electric shock may be stunned and remain unconscious for a considerable time. The violence of the shock may cause him to be hurled across a room or from a height and consequently to suffer other injuries as well. Lightning stroke may produce injuries in which bones are split along their lengths and the tissues rent as though by an explosion. On the other hand, it may leave the person physically unharmed.

The heart is sometimes brought at once to a standstill and the patient dies. Compressing the heart may restore a normal beat; in other cases it may keep the patient alive until ventricular fibrillation can be stopped by the appropriate machine (*see* page 23) but in other cases again the heart may have been damaged beyond recovery so that all efforts to revive the victim are unavailing. Sometimes the heart continues to beat, but perhaps imperceptibly. Respiration may stop because of the effect of the current on the brain and the only hope of recovery in such a case lies in artificial ventilation (*see* Chapter 2). The usual precautions against the rescuer's being electrocuted must, of course, be taken.

Local effects

The usual cause is direct contact of some part of the body with a source of electricity. The effects may be the result of the electricity or the heat or both, as when the element of an electric fire is touched. Heat is also generated if a flash occurs and if flammable objects catch fire. Sometimes there is only a small, blackened puncture mark, sometimes there is an area of shrunken, hard, yellow skin or of actual charring. Such burns are always deep and may be very deep indeed. A child that grasps the bar of an electric fire may suffer destruction of skin, fat and tendons. The full extent of death of the tissues is not easy to determine and it often happens that after obviously dead tissues have been cut

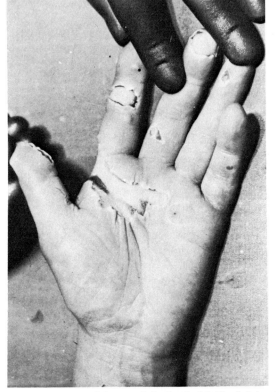

*Figure 7.7. Electrical burns of the hand. (a) The left hand
became moderately scarred*

away more tissues are found later to have succumbed so that bones
become exposed and joints open (*Figure 7.7*). Burns caused by heat
have the effects already described.

A phenomenon that is sometimes seen is purplish-brown marks
following the subcutaneous veins in the region of electrical injuries.

Irradiation

In serious cases the patient wastes from disorder of the bowel and
eventually dies from infection or aplastic anaemia owing to destruction
of the bone marrow. Failing its complete destruction, the marrow may
be induced to produce the abnormal cells of leukaemia. This is of no
practical importance to First Aid workers but what is important is that

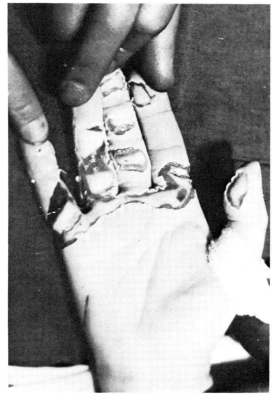

Figure 7.7(b). The burns on the right hand do not appear to be much more severe than those on the left hand, but in fact they were and they resulted in the loss of two fingers

the explosion of large-scale nuclear reactions produces enormous quantities of heat and flash burns may be extensive and severe.

Local effects resemble mild burns at first; they are rarely seen now but were all too common in the early days of radiotherapy. The danger of these injuries lies first in their initial mildness and secondly in the slowly progressive death or scarring of tissues, which may ultimately show malignant change. There is nothing that First Aid can do except to try and avoid infection and to arrange for medical care without delay.

Chemical burns

Chemical burns owe their effects to the destruction of the tissues by a chemical reaction between them and the injurious substance and also because the chemicals may be hot. The most urgent needs are to remove the harmful chemical and, if possible, to neutralize any that cannot be removed. The hazards of various industrial processes are well known and, when possible, appropriate facilities for treatment are provided and publicized in the factories and workshops concerned so that the injured person or his mates can take the first steps in treatment without delay.

Apart from the local effects, chemicals may be absorbed and cause widespread and sometimes fatal effects by their action on regions at a distance or by a general derangement of metabolism. Transfer of these patients to a Burns Unit is urgently necessary.

Alkalis

The main dangers come from the hydroxides of sodium, potassium, calcium and ammonium because these readily dissociate in solution and liberate high concentrations of hydroxyl ions; it is these that exert the caustic action from which some of these chemicals take their popular names. Because they are readily soluble, copious irrigation from any convenient source of water is good treatment. Any deposit or particles of caustic matter should be removed with something other than the bare fingers and this can be done while irrigation is being carried out.

Absorption does not occur in these cases.

Acids

The strong mineral acids such as hydrochloric, sulphuric and nitric corrode the tissues because of their ability to liberate hydrogen ions. Absorption does not occur and local treatment by copious irrigation suffices.

Because acids neutralize alkalis and vice versa it is often recommended that the one be used to treat burns caused by the other. Chemical neutralization is something of a refinement and need not be attempted if plenty of water is available.

Contaminated clothing should not be handled with the bare fingers but it must be removed as a matter of urgency. It may be possible to immerse the burnt part, but clothing must still be removed at once.

Where there are known chemical hazards of this type a buffer solution should be provided. This contains salts that are themselves harmless but ionize in opposite ways and are thereby enabled to 'mop up' hydroxyl or hydrogen ions equally well.

Buffer solution

Potassium dihydrogen phosphate (KH_2PO_4) 70 g
Disodium hydrogen phosphate ($Na_2HPO_4.12H_2O$) 180 g
Water 850 ml

This solution is used undiluted and can be employed with complete safety on the skin, in the eyes and as a mouth-wash. If a large area has been burned it should first be thoroughly washed with plain water and the buffer solution used to moisten a dressing that is then applied as a compress. For small burns the amount of buffer solution available may be enough for both irrigation and a compress.

Other acids act differently. They hardly ionize at all and the buffer solution, though harmless, has no special value.

Phenol (carbolic acid)

This is absorbed and can poison the nervous system and the kidneys. Phenol also has a selective action on the nerves in the region with which it comes in contact and it invalidates the prick test because the epithelial cells may survive a concentration that renders the nerve-endings insensitive.

Copious irrigation and a moist compress suffice and the patient should be despatched to hospital immediately.

Chromic acid

This acts locally to produce ulceration and can also be absorbed and cause poisoning. Irrigation and a dressing suffice for First Aid and again transfer to hospital is urgent. The ulcers are often too small to require grafting; they have a reputation for healing slowly but if infection is prevented this is not so.

Fumes of chromic acid or solution of chromates can cause ulceration of the nose and poison the nervous system. The First Aider can do no more than remove the patient (with due precautions) from the noxious environment and treat unconsciousness should it occur.

Hydrofluoric acid

This is used in several industries; its dangers are well known to safety officers, nurses and doctors in the works that use it but protective measures may fail. The acid penetrates the tissues easily and causes severe necrosis that is much more extensive than the area burned might lead one to expect.

Gloves should be removed at once and the part liberally washed with water or a warm, saturated solution of sodium bicarbonate. A cream containing magnesium oxide in glycerol should be massaged in but these burns are excruciatingly painful at first. The pain passes off later as the skin and the nerves supplying it become destroyed. Calcium gluconate is an antidote that may be injected into the skin. Nails should be cut short or removed because otherwise hydrofluoric acid remains under the nail and leads to osteitis of the terminal phalanx. Even with prompt and proper treatment disastrous crippling of the hands can follow apparently mild burns.

Phosphorus

The dangerous form of phosphorus is yellow phosphorus, which oxidizes so rapidly when in contact with air that it ignites and causes thermal burns. The part should be doused with water and any remaining phosphorus removed with the fingers suitably protected. Immersion is a valuable immediate step in treatment and, if practicable, the clothing should be removed while the patient is still immersed. Otherwise the hands must be protected and contaminated clothing rendered harmless by drenching with water, or immersion, lest remaining phosphorus ignite again. Sodium bicarbonate has been recommended to neutralize phosphoric acid, which is formed from the phosphorus. One per cent copper sulphate solution may be applied once to turn any remaining particles of phosphorus into black copper phosphide; this can be more easily seen and removed. More than one application of copper sulphate may cause poisoning.

Other chemicals

Mercury, nickel and arsenic may be absorbed and damage the bone marrow and nervous system. First Aid is to treat the thermal burns immediately and arrange transfer to hospital where specific antidotes can be used.

Paraffin, petrol and trichlorethylene irritate the skin to the extent of blistering if it is in contact with it for some minutes. They do not destroy the skin unless hot or alight. The treatment is then the treatment of thermal burns. The important thing is to lie the victim down at once and to extinguish the flames with whatever is to hand; usually this is the First Aider's coat or jacket, but may be a carpet, curtains or bedclothes. Water may carry burning liquid with it as it runs away but it may be all that is available to douse the burning person. Immersion or a shower bath may be used if practicable. Sand is a safe extinguisher of flammable liquids but has the important disadvantage of keeping the lately burning and therefore hot remains of clothing against the skin. Should there be nothing else available sand may be used and the burnt person extricated from it immediately the flames are extinguished. The contamination of the burnt surface by sand that may be germ-ridden is regrettable but not unmanageable.

Chemical extinguishers may be used, bearing in mind that they will damage the eyes.

Where the risk of burning exists it would be a sensible precaution to train workmen as well as First Aiders to extinguish burning dummies and to supplement the customary extinguishers at key points with fireproof sheets in which to wrap victims of ignition.

Burns caused by chemicals without the complication of ignition are usually fairly localized and therefore rarely cause shock in the surgical sense, but as they may require early surgical treatment any 'primary shock', that is, emotional collapse or syncope, should not be treated with the traditional cup of tea. Provided that there is no inflammable vapour about there is no serious objection to a cigarette but it will have to be handled for the patient if his hands have suffered.

SUMMARY OF FIRST AID

Many First Aiders seem to become confused about the presence and treatment of shock when called upon to deal with a genuine burn. They are well aware of the fact that severe shock can occur and may require urgent treatment but 'Treat for shock' figures so prominently in their textbooks that they easily lose their sense of proportion and may refer trivial burns to hospital and impose all sorts of unnecessary restrictions on a patient and cause him great inconvenience.

Few really serious burns are seen by First Aiders. They are usually despatched to hospital at once by workmates or members of the family, before shock appears. Shock in the serious form that requires special treatment does not occur except with burns affecting about one-tenth or more of the surface of the body. Emotional shock, pain and mental distress do not come into the serious category.

Reduced to its simplest terms the treatment of thermal burns is:

1. Apply a clean or sterile covering.
2. Arrange medical care.
3. Allow nothing to be taken by mouth except with burns affecting about 10 per cent or more of the body.

Many burns are trivial, as from small splashes of hot liquids, fat and so forth, or from brief contact with flame or a hot body. The area burnt may be considerably smaller than a postage stamp. Whether there is blistering or not, burns of this size require no more than a good wash with soap and tap water followed by a dry dressing that should, if possible, remain undisturbed for a week or 10 days. Even if still unhealed another dressing is all that is required unless there are signs of spreading inflammation. Most of such burns are dealt with successfully by the patient or his companions and medical care is rarely required.

Burns the size of a stamp or larger and caused by molten metal, electricity or strong chemicals, need medical care after appropriate First Aid. They are usually deep and may qualify for primary excision and grafting, especially if they are on the hands or feet.

Whatever the apparent depth when first seen, burns affecting 0.5 per cent of the body's surface require medical attention (0.5 per cent is roughly half the area of the *patient's* palm and fingers).

Flame burns

1. If the clothing is alight lie the patient down and smother the flames with a suitable wrapping—blanket, rug or coat.
2. Do not remove clothing or adherent matter.
3. Wrap in a clean cloth or sheet.
4. Send to hospital.
5. Drinks are permissible because these burns are almost always extensive enough to cause shock.

Hot water burns

1. If seen *at once*, hot wet clothing should be removed; it can act as a poultice and aggravate the damage.
2. Otherwise treat as for flame burns.

Electrical burns

1. Remove the patient from the current (taking suitable precautions) or switch off the current.
2. If breathing is not perceptible (*a*) ensure a clear air passage and (*b*) carry out artificial ventilation. It may be necessary to squeeze the heart as well.
3. When breathing has been resumed look for and treat (*a*) wounds; (*b*) fractures; and (*c*) burns.

Chemical burns

Local treatment

1. Remove contaminated clothing at once.
2. Irrigate freely with water; this includes immersion and the use of a shower bath if practicable.
3. Apply the appropriate antidote if available but do not waste time looking for or making one.
   (*a*) Mineral acids and strong alkalis: buffer solution (*see* page 165).
   (*b*) Hydrofluoric acid: magnesium oxide paste massaged in and calcium gluconate compresses.
   (*c*) Phosphorus: sodium bicarbonate may be used but copper sulphate solution is better avoided.

General treatment

Apart from recognizing that extensive chemical burns cause shock, the First Aider has no remedy except to carry out artificial ventilation and cardiac massage should they be necessary. The use of specific antidotes such as dimercaprol for poisoning by mercury, nickel, arsenic, and so on, and the treatment of damage to the kidneys, marrow and nervous system are skilled medical tasks.

Complicated burns

Fractures and other injuries should be treated as circumstances require but with the need to give priority to treatment of shock always in mind.

Burns in difficult circumstances

The above measures may be applied equally well in primitive and civilized communities provided that skilled medical care is readily available. If the patient is out of easy reach of medical care drinking should be encouraged, provided that large quantities are not given all at once. Very large quantities may be required but the individual drinks should be suitably spaced. The urine passed should be kept, if possible, so that its quantity can be measured and its composition studied if required. A free flow of clear urine—1.2—2.0 litres (2—4 pints) in 24 hours, that is, 30 ml (1 oz) or more an hour—is reassuring. Scanty or bloody urine is a serious sign, but even if the flow should cease altogether drinking should continue in an attempt to replace the liquid seeping out of the circulation.

If the patient vomits, drinks should be withheld for a while and then tried again cautiously. Intravenous infusion is vitally necessary because vomiting may be the result of shock and stop only when shock has been controlled.

If the choice should have to be made between moving a severely burnt person a short distance to a cottage hospital, dispensary or other place of scanty medical attention and sending him on a journey of 2 or 3 hours to a place where full facilities exist, it should be remembered that the seriously burnt travel best at once, before shock has become fully established.

In hot climates cover is desirable to keep off dust and insects but the covering should be light. In cold places warmth should be retained by adding extra layers of covers. If the temperature can be taken this is a valuable precaution against hyperpyrexia. A temperature above $102°F$ $(39°C)$ should be reduced to $99°-100°F$ $(37.2-37.7°C)$ by removing covers, moistening dressings by clean or boiled water, fanning and the use of aspirin in doses of 0.3, 0.6 or 1.0 g (according to age) every 2—3 hours as required.

If penicillin is available 1 million units may be injected into an unburnt fleshy area but antibacterial substances should not be applied to the burnt area except in definitive treatment.

8

HEAD INJURIES

Head injuries are often understood to mean injuries affecting the brain-box or cranium and its contents, but it is better to include all injuries above the neck because there is much in common between cranio-cerebral injury and injury affecting the facial skeleton as a whole. Furthermore, the two types of injury may occur together.

CRANIOCEREBRAL INJURIES

Craniocerebral injuries are dominated by the presence of damage to the brain and the possibility that it will suffer from the effects of com-plications, particularly hypoxia, bleeding and infection.

Broadly speaking, the brain may be damaged by violence applied directly, as by penetration or compression, or transmitted by the impact of the bony ledges of the skull and the dural partitions within it (*Figure 8.1*).

The manner and nature of cerebral damage

Direct violence

The damaging effects of penetration need no elaboration. They vary from the superficial disruption caused by a depressed fracture to extensive pulping caused by the passage of a missile or other object.

Intracranial pressure

Perhaps the most important pressure within the skull is the perfusion pressure, which is the difference between the pressure in the arteries to the brain and the pressure within the skull. It is now possible to measure directly the pressure within the skull and this has shown that previous ideas about it were in many cases wrong. For example, if the pressure within the spinal cord is measured (by lumbar puncture) it

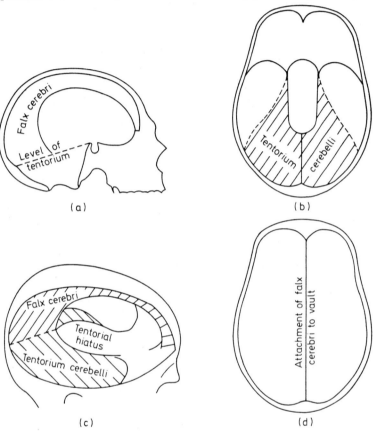

Figure 8.1. The ledges and partitions within the skull: (a) from side; (b) from above; (c) obliquely from above; and (d) the under surface of the vault of the skull

bears no reliable relationship to the pressure within the skull and it is also clear that the signs that were believed to signify a rise in intra-cranial pressure can occur without it or be absent when the pressure is raised. Other important additions to First Aiders' knowledge are the facts that the simple action of turning the head to one side can ob-struct the veins sufficiently to raise the pressure within the skull and that any straining or choking, such as occurs particularly in an epileptic fit, produces a dramatic rise. It will be readily understood that if the pressure exerted on the brain goes up without any corresponding rise in the arterial pressure to the brain, the perfusion pressure will fall with the result that the brain is deprived of some of the oxygen-carrying blood of which it may be in urgent need.

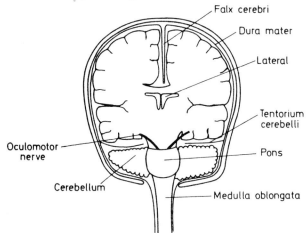

Figure 8.2. The brain-stem passes through a gap in a horizontal membrane (the tentorium cerebelli) that separates the cerebrum, above, from the cerebellum below

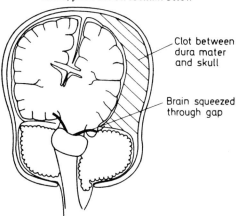

Figure 8.3. Displacement of the brain can cause some of it to be squeezed through the gap and press on blood vessels and the constrictor nerve to the pupil of the eye

The rise in intracranial pressure usually occurs in association with more or less distortion of the brain, particularly where the brain-stem passes through the gap in the tentorium cerebelli (*Figure 8.2*). A part of the brain that rests on the upper surface of the tentorium can be displaced into the gap beside the brain-stem so that the edge of this structure bulges downwards. This is known as tentorial herniation and it has two important effects (*Figure 8.3*). One is that it presses on the 3rd cranial nerve, which runs through the gap, and so paralyzes the sympathetic nerve fibres that are responsible for constricting the pupil of the eye, which consequently dilates to a degree that reflects the pressure exerted on the nerve. If both pupils are found to be widely dilated and fixed there is severe pressure being exerted by tentorial herniation on both sides, and on the brain-stem itself, so that the outlook is very grave.

The second important effect is that the pressure on the herniated part of the brain that is normally above the tentorium cerebelli damages the blood supply to an important region nearby. It is now well recognized that many of the lasting effects of head injury, as well as deaths, are the result not of the initial damage, or primary lesions, but of the secondary lesions caused by swelling, distortion and interference with the blood supply of parts of the brain. The importance of any event that raises intracranial pressure, cuts down blood supply or reduces the oxygen supply to the brain will add further to these damaging effects and needs no further explanation. Blue lips mean a blue brain and a blue brain is suffering damage that may be widespread and permanent with disastrous consequences for the patient and his family.

Indirect violence

It is well known that a boxer can render his opponent unconscious by striking him on the jaw, that is, without applying force directly upon the brain-box. The explanation has been provided by experiments in which a known force has been applied to different parts of the head in different circumstances. From these experiments it was found that it made a great difference whether the head was fixed or was free to move. With the head firmly fixed, a certain force had no effect upon the consciousness of the subject but when the head was free to move that same force, applied to the same place, could induce unconsciousness. Even when the head was free to move, however, the concussive effect depended upon the site of impact and it was realized that what was important was not whether the head could move but whether it did move, and in an appropriate way, when struck.

The head is supported upon the neck by joints that allow it to swing back and forth or from side to side and also to twist. A blow upon the top of the head and directed down the axis of the neck may simply cram the cervical joints together momentarily and discomfort the victim without disturbing consciousness. If that same blow is directed elsewhere on the head it will pass by one or other axis of movement of the head upon the neck and set it suddenly in motion about that axis. Unconsciousness may result. The determining influence is the speed with which the head is set in motion or, if already moving, brought to rest.

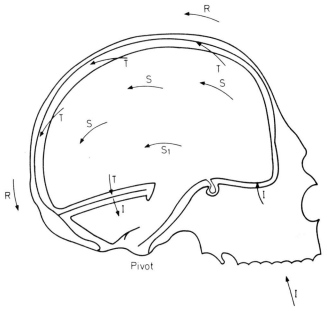

Figure 8.4. Forces acting within the skull and strains resulting. R: Rotation; T: Tension; S: Shearing; I: Impact

The effects of rapid acceleration or deceleration of the head are exerted upon the brain by ledges and partitions within the skull. A blow upon the point of the jaw, for example, sets the head swinging sharply backwards. The skull starts to move a fraction of a second before the brain, which can be regarded as floating in a water cushion of cerebrospinal fluid, and the floor of the anterior fossa strikes the juxtaposed surface of the brain and damages it (*Figure 8.4 I*). The horizontal partition of the tentorium cerebelli moves with the skull and consequently strikes the upper surface of the cerebellum (*Figure 8.4 I*). These are forces of impact. At the same time the floor of the posterior fossa moves downwards and momentarily away from the cerebellum so that there is a sudden traction or suction effect between them (*Figure 8.4 T*). This also can cause damage. By the time that the skull has been brought to rest the brain may have attained a fairly high speed and it in turn will be brought to rest, but by impact against the skull and its partitions. Thus the initial impacts become tractions and vice versa and more damage may be inflicted upon the brain.

These are not the only injurious forces and it is now known that distortion of the brain caused by shearing stresses within it is of great importance. From *Figure 8.4* it will be appreciated that as the skull moves relative to the brain it will in some places be moving neither towards nor away from it but past it (*Figure 8.4 S*) and the vessels connecting the skull and the brain will transmit the motion of the one

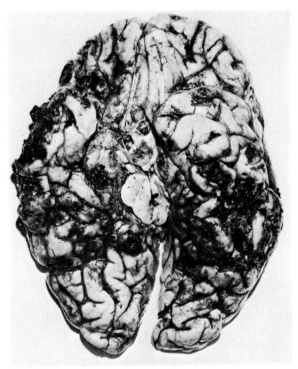

Figure 8.5. Undersurface of brain
(By courtesy of S. Sevitt)

to the other (and perhaps be injured in the process). The surface of the brain first receives the pull, which is then transmitted to the deeper structures (*Figure 8.4 S*). Because the sponge-like brain can be deformed the transmission of these forces is a relatively gradual process that entails the drag of layer upon layer right down to the region of the brain-stem, which acts as a pivot and itself suffers deformation (*Figure 8.4 S_1*).

When the brain of the victim of a fatal head injury is examined it may show extensive pulping (*Figure 8.5*). This is usually most striking in an area adjoining the point of impact (coup lesion) and another roughly diametrically opposite (contre-coup lesion). On the other hand, the brain and the skull may appear undamaged to the naked eye and it is then presumed that imperceptible lesions owing to various forces have caused death. Such lesions may be present elsewhere in brains that show pulping of opposite poles. One of the interesting things about such injuries is that the severe pulping is not fatal and that the patient that dies of his head injury is usually killed by the much smaller areas and degrees of damage in vital regions such as the brain-stem and by the secondary effects such as swelling.

Compression of the brain

Any injury of the brain causes more or less swelling and with the more serious injuries this can become the most important consequence. 'Swelling' is preferable to 'oedema' because the swollen injured brain has more or less bruising and not merely an excess of liquid within it, as in true oedema.

Unlike the obvious and immediate effects of direct and indirect violence, cerebral compression exerts its effects subtly. A well known but less frequent cause than swelling is the accumulation of blood upon the surface of the brain or within its substance. It is tempting to regard this as exerting its effects by an actual rise of pressure, such as may be caused by pressing one's fingers upon an inflated balloon. In fact, the brain is more like a sponge and the substance of the sponge is represented by the neural tissues. These are permeated by the actual spaces of the blood vessels and the ventricular system and by the potential spaces that ramify from the subarachnoid space and penetrate the fine structure of the cerebral tissues.

When pressure is applied to a sponge filled with water it becomes indented at the site of pressure because water is displaced. In the case of the brain the liquid displaced by pressure can be accommodated partly by the absorption of cerebrospinal fluid and partly by the movement of blood out of the unyielding skull into the vessels of the neck and face. There may, therefore, be no measurable rise of pressure within the brain-box. In this case the signs and symptoms that result are to be explained by distortion of the brain and by obstruction of the circulation in the distorted part. The nerve cells are especially sensitive to lack of oxygen, which soon follows any impediment to the blood supply.

This is not to deny that an actual rise of pressure takes place nor to suggest that such a rise plays no part in the symptoms and signs of cerebral injury. An enlarging mass can obstruct the flow of blood by pressing on large vessels and by pressure or distortion it can block the narrow parts of the ventricular system (*Figure 8.6*). The cerebrospinal fluid cannot then pass from its sources within the brain to be absorbed

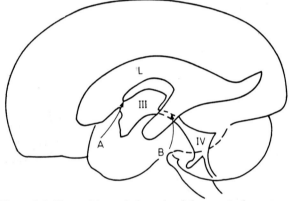

Figure 8.6. The cavities and channels of the ventricular system. A and B are isthmuses, liable to be blocked by pressure or distortion. L: Lateral ventricle (paired). III and IV: 3rd and 4th ventricles (paired)

in the arachnoid granulations upon the brain's surface. The pressure within the ventricular system will rise (and be transmitted throughout the brain-box) to the pressure exerted by the secretory process, which will then cease.

The cause of unconsciousness

In the past unconsciousness has been regarded as being the result of depression of cerebral function as a whole. It was well known that localized damage, whether severe and amounting to laceration or nothing worse than mild contusion, was often associated with unconsciousness.

It was also well known that unconsciousness could be present without any visible damage in the brain. Because of the occurrence of a blow the cause was ascribed to a diffuse shaking up of the brain (commotio cerebri), from which belief the term concussion was derived.

The present concepts of cerebral injury accord well with recent studies that have shown the importance of the basal regions of the brain for the control of consciousness. A rather loose network of cells and fibres (whence the name reticular formation) has long been known as part of the microscopic structure of the upper end of the brain-stem and the adjoining basal regions of the brain itself. This reticular formation is now accorded the role of driver of the cerebral cortex; activity within the reticular formation stimulates activity within the cerebral cortex and artificial stimulation of the basal area will rouse a sleeping animal, whereas stimulation of the cortex alone will not. Small destructive lesions in the reticular formation can cause permanent disturbance of consciousness but large amounts of cortex can be removed without influencing it at all.

The fact that the region occupied by the reticular formation is a pivot upon which the brain can swing makes it especially vulnerable to any event that sets the brain suddenly in motion or brings it suddenly to rest, and it has been shown by high speed cinematography that a blow on the head can also cause a sinuous crumpling of the brain-stem. Any other disturbance of this area, as by pressure or reduced supply of blood or oxygen, can also cause unconsciousness.

Some reasons why severe destructive injuries of the brain may never dull consciousness are now clear. Unless there has been a sudden acceleration or deceleration of the skull and brain the reticular formation can escape unscathed. Soldiers have been shot through the head and protested when forbidden to fight on; men have had their heads crushed and heard the bone break without losing consciousness.

Fractures of the brain-box

Fractures of the skull are not necessarily serious. They become so when the broken bone injures the brain, when the force that causes fracture also causes damage to the brain, or when a blood vessel is torn. Fractures are also important when there is a breach of the structures between the meninges and the air—either the general atmosphere or the air in the cavities within the skull.

Fractures and bleeding

In First Aid teaching and practice particular emphasis is laid upon cerebral compression as a sequel of head injury. This can occur with or without fracture, and bleeding upon the surface of the brain or within its substance is one of the more simply understandable causes, though much less frequent than the swelling that has already been described (*see* page 177). The best known source of surface bleeding is the middle meningeal artery but in fact any of the meningeal vessels, arteries or veins, may be torn and the bleeding occurs either between the skull and the dura mater (extradural) or deep to it (subdural). In the former instance the vessels may be torn by a fracture across the grooves that they occupy in the bone. They can also be torn by the separation of dura from bone that occurs when the skull is deformed by impact.

Subdural bleeding is caused by the tearing of vessels running between the brain and the dura mater that occurs when the skull moves suddenly past the brain or away from it (*Figure 8.4*). It also accompanies surface pulping of the brain.

Intracerebral haemorrhage is owing to direct or indirect damage to the brain and may be facilitated by disease of the blood vessels.

These types of intracranial haemorrhage can occur separately or in various combinations and as far as First Aid is concerned there is no distinction between them. Indeed, there is no justification for attempting to distinguish between a natural cerebral vascular accident and intracranial haemorrhage caused by injury. In each case the patient is likely to become unconscious and may or may not show signs of injury to the head.

Depressed fractures

The various sorts of depression are not themselves necessarily of any great importance but there are two important possibilities with depressed fractures. They can cause bleeding or damage to the brain and they may be open. Closed depressions may be recognizable by palpation and very shortly after injury a palpable dent can confidently be ascribed to a depressed fracture. An hour or so later, however, blood beneath the scalp has begun to congeal and the edges of the effusion feel firm while the centre is still soft and impressionable. A clot can mimic a depression in the skull very closely. In the early stages a dent should be regarded seriously but if a day or more has passed and the patient is well without having been unconscious or having bled from the facial apertures a dent that can be felt need not be regarded with the same urgency.

Open fractures

Whatever their nature these are serious because they carry the risk of infection. This risk is especially great with open depressed fractures because hair or other contaminated material is often trapped in the fracture line. It is also likely that the depressed bone will have torn the dura mater or perhaps penetrated a large venous channel. The fracture may be visible through a wound in the scalp and although there may be little visible indentation it may be that the inner table of the skull has been more extensively broken and more deeply depressed than the outer (*Figure 8.7*). For this reason any fracture visible in a scalp wound is an emergency irrespective of the patient's state of consciousness.

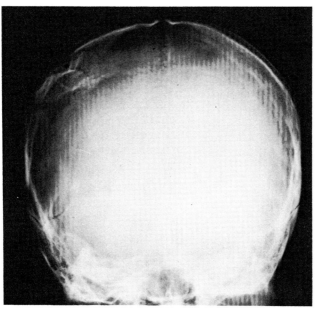

Figure 8.7. Depressed fracture, showing the greater displacement of the inner table

Fractures of the base of the skull usually declare themselves by bleeding from the nose, ears or mouth or by bruising in the eyelids and under the conjunctiva. Such bleeding may come from nothing more serious than injury of the nose, ears or mouth without any breach of the meninges, but the escape of watery blood or a blood-stained watery liquid leaves no doubt that the meningeal barrier has been torn. Again, suspicion that the meninges have been torn calls for urgent treatment whether the patient is unconscious or not.

Late effects of head injury

The late effects of head injury are beyond the scope of First Aid but will be considered briefly because they may be disproportionate to the state in which the First Aider finds the patient and important practical considerations spring from this fact. A patient at first fully conscious and even without any gap in his memory of events may have suffered serious damage to the brain and come to require urgent surgical treatment. On the other hand, a state of desperate gravity can be followed by a complete and rapid recovery if dealt with correctly in the first place.

With modern methods of resuscitation and treatment it has become possible to save the lives of persons who have suffered injury of the brain that will leave them permanently and pitiably crippled in mind or body. Parts of the brain concerned with intellectual, emotional and physical activity may be irrecoverably damaged while parts governing vital functions escape unscathed or, though injured, can recover if given time to do so by keeping the patient alive by more or less artificial means. The First Aider can be grateful for being relieved of the responsibility for the ultimate decisions about how to handle these tragic victims of accident.

Unconsciousness

Unconsciousness has not been satisfactorily defined but it is often said to be easily recognizable and the most dramatic consequence of head injury. In fact, however, what is being observed is responsiveness; this is not quite the same as unconsciousness because responsiveness may carry awareness and memory whereas unconsciousness does not. In practice the distinction may not be made until afterwards and it may be agreed that at the time there is no need to make the distinction. Nevertheless, although it is more accurate to use the word responsiveness, this is so unfamiliar to First Aiders, and others, that there is less likely to be confusion if the more familiar but less accurate word unconsciousness is used. It is fundamentally a sign of impairment of the activity of more or less of the brain and may result from many causes other than injury of the head. With the present high speed travel on the roads many parts of the body are liable to be injured at the same time and although the head may figure prominently among these injuries the unconscious state may have other causes.

Apart from the possibly purely mechanical effects of distortion, damage to the brain causes unconsciousness because in one way or another the supply of blood and oxygen is reduced below the level required to allow nerve cells to function normally. Pressure exerted locally, by swelling or through the cranium can cause this. Equally, the vital oxygen supply can be reduced below the critical level if there is not enough blood in circulation to bring it to the brain or if the concentration of oxygen in the blood reaching the brain is inadequate. The three conditions may also combine to cause unconsciousness although none of them in isolation would have done so.

The First Aid worker must, therefore, be on the lookout for other injuries that may be contributing to unconsciousness but masked by its presence. The conditions to be borne prominently in mind are oligaemic shock and damage to the chest and its contents.

Anaemic hypoxia

Generally speaking, the victim of head injury alone does not present the classical picture of established shock. If there is manifest shock a search should be made for other injuries capable of causing serious bleeding but whether other injuries are found or not the urgency appropriate to the head injury is increased if shock is present. The reduced oxygen supply that is liable to accompany oligaemic shock may tip the balance disastrously against recovery of the nerve cells in the brain and prompt resuscitation should be aimed at.

Hypoxic hypoxia

This is even more important because it frequently occurs and in most cases it can be dealt with effectually by the First Aider. It is, however, all too often ignored or not recognized.

Obstructed breathing

This is much more often present and is much more easy to overlook than is generally realized. Usually textbooks of First Aid lay proper emphasis on keeping the air passage clear but this is not an easy subject to teach realistically without having an unconscious patient as a subject. References to the stertorous breathing that accompanies unconsciousness have little to say about its immediate cause, its importance or the way in which to relieve it. It cannot be emphasized too strongly that noisy breathing must be regarded as obstructed breathing. It may be that

snoring is such a familiar feature of the sleep of some persons in perfect
health (and a subject for humour) that snoring by an unconscious
person is not regarded as important. Snoring is a sign that breathing is
impeded. The sleeping snorer has his protective reflexes intact and these
guard him against a serious degree of obstruction but the reflexes of
the victim of head injury may be gravely depressed and offer no protection whatsoever against increasing respiratory obstruction and
consequent cerebral hypoxia.

Another type of stertorous breathing is caused by blood, cerebrospinal fluid, regurgitated food, accumulated sputum or displaced false
teeth obstructing the upper air passages. Strident or wheezy breathing
also means obstruction, but the deep gasping respiration that sometimes
accompanies unconsciousness does not. However, no harm will come to
the person with such breathing if he is treated as though he were
obstructed and the rule 'noisy breathing is obstructed breathing' can
safely be taught without exception.

Froth on the lips is popularly associated with madness, rage and
epilepsy, but it too is a sign of obstructed breathing.

Cyanosis has many causes but the efficient cause is a reduced amount
of oxyhaemoglobin in the blood. The most frequent cause is defective
oxygenation but this may be for several reasons, such as inadequate
oxygen in the inspired air or reduced ventilation, which reduces the
normal movements of oxygen into and carbon dioxide out of the
lungs; obstruction to the passage of gases through the tissues between
blood and air in the lungs and also obstructed passage of blood through
the vessels in the lungs. Heart failure, poisoning and some drugs also
cause cyanosis but need not be considered here.

Mild cyanosis is easily overlooked in the dark-skinned even in
favourable circumstances while poor illumination and discoloration
of the face by dirt, smoke and the like can mask markedly blue lips
and ears. Cyanosis may then be recognized in the finger-nails, the
skin generally, or the lining of the mouth or eyelids. It occasionally
happens that a victim of head injury has bruised lips, but even if this
were mistaken for cyanosis no harm would result.

Cyanosis arising from damage to the thoracic cage and its contents
will be dealt with in Chapter 9. It is enough to say here that cyanosis
with noisy breathing, whether or not there is froth on the lips, is
most likely to be caused by respiratory obstruction and that steps should
at once be taken to relieve the obstruction. Cyanosis with easy breathing
suggests other causes.

These three signs of obstructed breathing are well known but in
practice it is remarkable how often First Aiders either fail to notice
them or fail to recognize the urgent need for treatment. It should,

therefore, be impressed upon them that the unconscious patient, whatever the cause of his unconsciousness, must be assured of a clear air passage and that this applies whether the signs of obstruction are present or not. The signs must be sought in every unconscious patient and when they are present they demand instant attention. Quite apart from the dangers to the respiratory organs, obstructed breathing causes hypoxia that can seriously aggravate existing damage to the brain. Physical damage that may itself be completely recoverable can interfere with the respiratory centre in the brain-stem, lead to hypoxia and so cause further and perhaps irreparable harm to nerve cells that are literally in danger of their very lives. Blue lips are accompanied by a blue brain. This danger exists at all ages but is especially grave in old persons, whom mild or transient hypoxia can change from alert and interested persons into doddering and demented burdens on their kin.

Hypoxia is not only one of the consequences of unconsciousness but may be the cause of it.

Head and other injuries in combination

The combination of head and other injuries is a frequent result of road accidents. When a vehicle stops suddenly, unless the occupants are restrained by correctly fitted and designed safety belts they are thrown violently forwards against wind-screen, dashboard, steering wheel or front seats. The head, face, chest, abdomen and limbs may be injured in any combination. Pedestrians and cyclists are liable to similar combined and serious injuries.

It is usually obvious that serious injuries have occurred but it may be extremely difficult to recognize just what they are and what part the separate injuries play in producing the state in which the victim is found. Unconsciousness may result from severe bleeding, which has caused anaemic cerebral hypoxia; from damage to the chest, heart or lungs, causing hypoxic cerebral hypoxia, or from head injury. These three causes may all be present at once and each responsible in part for the unconsciousness, but it is important to remember that although the head has suffered obvious injury the cause of accompanying unconsciousness may be elsewhere and must be sought. It should also be remembered that a blow on the head can seriously injure the neck. This is particularly likely to happen if the face or brow is struck because such a force can cause fracture by hyperextension (*Figure 8.8*). Although it is rare, this sort of injury should be borne in mind when it is intended to clear the air passages by tilting the head well back; lifting the jaw forward with a thumb in the mouth is safer.

The unconscious patient cannot complain of pain, he may be restless and difficult to examine, he may even move broken or dislocated limbs as freely as uninjured ones. The signs of other injuries may be masked because of damage to the brain but the signs of shock suggest very

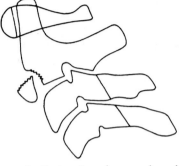

Figure 8.8. Avulsion fracture of the body of C2 caused by a blow on the brow that snapped the head back hard

strongly that serious haemorrhage has occurred. Head injury alone does not cause the signs of established shock but it can abolish the pain, tenderness or rigidity that would direct the examiner's attention to the abdomen or pelvis, where the shock has perhaps originated.

The difficulties that can arise are exemplified by the case quoted in Chapter 2. The First Aider cannot be expected to analyse complexities of that kind but he can be taught to recognize and treat what lies within his power. His efforts may be unavailing because the injuries are fatal but those efforts must be made. The main needs may be obvious; they must be met in the hope that success will follow.

Unconsciousness increases the difficulties of diagnosing injuries and it may cause serious medical conditions to be completely overlooked unless a third person provides relevant information. Safeguards such as cards warning that the patient suffers from a particular disease or is taking certain drugs should always be sought because of their sometimes vital importance to diagnosis and treatment. A more general warning of possibly dangerous drugs and disorders is provided by the Medic Alert* Bracelet (*Figure 8.9*), which has appropriate information on its back and should be known to all First Aiders.

Degrees of unconsciousness

It has long been customary to grade unconsciousness into confusion, stupor and coma, but no matter how these states be defined the

*Details of membership may be obtained from 9 Hanover Street, London W1R 9HF

definitions will ignore the variations within these states and tend to discourage attention to important manifestations.

Sherrington's experiments about the turn of the century led him to recognize the nervous system as an integrative agent. Its complex organization and its detailed functional relationship with all other

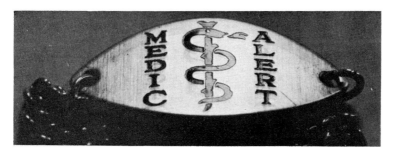

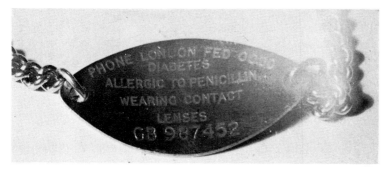

Figure 8.9. The two surfaces of the Medic Alert disc and bracelet

parts of the organism enable it to adjust the activity of any or all of the organism's components to effective changes in the surroundings. Injury of the brain impairs more or less the ability of the organism to respond with biological propriety to environmental change.

With modern methods of treatment the victim with head injuries that were previously of fatal or crippling consequence may now recover if his injuries are recognized and dealt with promptly. It therefore becomes important to acquaint the First Aider with the fact that confusion, stupor and coma are not simply three states of increasing gravity but that they are three arbitrary sections of a continuous range of varied integration, or responsiveness, of the victim of head injury. The progress from 'confusion' to 'stupor' or from 'stupor' to 'coma' is of great importance and it may represent a mortal deterioration. What should also be recognized is that deterioration within these states is a sign that urgent measures are more urgently required lest shortly no measure will afford relief.

Recovery is reassuring and might seem, therefore, to deserve less emphasis than deterioration. The two processes are, however, opposite expressions of the same thing—a change in the level of consciousness—and the First Aider must be alert to observe change in either direction.

Confusion

This leaves the patient able to understand and to reply when spoken to but the clarity of his understanding and the appositeness of his reply should be tested, and repeatedly. If at first the patient can give an account of himself but later can do no more than give his name and age, staring blankly around at people and things that he previously recognized, he must be presumed to have worsened. The manner of the reply may be as informative as the reply itself. The fact that a patient can be roused and urged to answer simple questions is the reverse of reassuring if he previously answered them promptly and without their being repeated.

Stupor

This deprives the patient of his ability to frame answers, and he may merely grunt or mutter when disturbed by questions or examination. Again, the manner as well as the nature of the response is noteworthy. A mildly painful stimulus such as pressure on the supra-orbital notch, behind the jaw or on the tendo Achillis is useful. In light stupor the head or foot will be purposefully withdrawn and if not incapacitated by injury the patient will use his hand to remove the offending stimulus. In deep stupor there may be no more than an ineffective grimace or a shrugging of the shoulders; neither is directed obviously towards disposing of the stimulus and these responses indicate a less successfully integrated response. A change from one stage to the other is significant.

Coma

In coma, the patient merely stiffens his limbs or makes no response at all to any stimulus and is in grave and immediate danger.

In summary it may be said that it would be preferable if the terms confusion, stupor and coma were not used and if First Aiders and others were encouraged to record their tests and the patient's responses. Perhaps a more practicable course is to adopt the gradation of the ambulance report form recommended by the Department of Health. This offers normal consciousness, the ability to answer questions, the ability to carry out simple actions on request and unconsciousness. These four grades should be easily and reliably distinguishable and variations within these grades should also be recognizable.

Lucid interval

This period of more or less consciousness intervening between two periods of unconsciousness is one of the classical signs of intracranial bleeding, and the fact that it occurs makes it very important that a person who has recovered consciousness after head injury should be kept under observation. Any subsequent deterioration in the level of consciousness is of grave importance, as, indeed, is any deterioration from whatever level of consciousness.

These observations are of great value and form the basis of skilled medical care, because it is upon the improvement or deterioration in the state of consciousness that the nature and timing of treatment is decided in hospital. It may be objected that it is sufficient for the First Aider to be taught the three customary stages of impairment of consciousness and to recognize their degree of gravity. This objection is not valid.

First, it is very helpful to the doctor who receives the patient to know if his condition has altered and in what way. If he can be given a reliable account of what the patient has said or done, and how, he will be that much better informed than by a bald label of coma, stupor or confusion. Even if the First Aider cannot spontaneously provide a clear picture of what has happened, if he has been taught that careful and repeated observation is important his answers to the doctor's questions are quite likely to elucidate the course of events.

Second, there may be several injured persons to deal with and those with some knowledge of First Aid may have to decide who needs priority in treatment. Unconsciousness shares immediate priority with obstructed breathing and severe shock. An open fracture of the tibia is dramatic and more amenable than unconsciousness to the active measures described in First Aid manuals but the victim is in less urgent need of conveyance to hospital. The patient whose level of consciousness is deteriorating should be moved to hospital before a patient who is improving. This is not to suggest that decisions are easily reached in all cases. What is to be the choice when circumstances demand that it be made between a person who is confused and is deteriorating and another who is already in coma? The First Aider cannot be accurately and infallibly guided in such a dilemma but he should not be deprived of the knowledge of signs and symptoms that may guide him in less difficult circumstances.

Stress has been laid upon these general changes in the condition of the unconscious person because they are important. The local signs such as the size and equality of the pupils and the nature of the breathing are also important but it is not sufficient to note these while ignoring the general signs.

Fits

Convulsions of one kind or another sometimes occur in association with head injury and indeed may be responsible for it. They can start at any time after the moment of injury and generally speaking their significance becomes increasingly serious with the delay in onset. Fits starting within a short time of injury are most often seen in children and may mean nothing more than that the injury has for the time being irritated part of the brain. Complete recovery often occurs. Fits starting days or weeks after injury usually mean that part of the brain has suffered lasting damage and the fits may occur from time to time throughout the patient's life.

Apart from the standard First Aid it is important to note the course of events. One part of the body, often one side of the mouth, starts to twitch, the movements may spread and become more vigorous until the whole body is jerking. Breathing is stertorous and froth appears on the lips, which become blue, as does the brain. It is not usually possible to relieve this condition because the cause is the spasm of the muscles. Fortunately breathing usually reverts to normal as the fit subsides but it is wise then to clear the mouth and throat. The place at which the fits start should be noted and also the direction of spread for this may be helpful in diagnosis. While a fit is in progress, First Aiders will usually be better engaged in observing its cause and removing any hazards than in possibly damaging attempts to restrain the patient. Fits must be regarded as increasing the need for urgent medical attention, because the period of hypoxia, indicated by cyanosis, can add seriously to any existing damage to the brain.

THE TREATMENT OF CRANIOCEREBRAL INJURIES

Treatment of craniocerebral injuries centres on the care of the air passages, treatment of wounds and bleeding and the management of other injuries, if present. Apart from trying to protect it from hypoxia, the First Aider can do nothing to treat the injured brain but he can render valuable service by his reports and his efforts to prevent further damage.

The care of the air passages

If the patient is unconscious the following steps should be taken whether the breathing is obviously obstructed or not. If there is obvious obstruction it must receive priority in treatment because it shares with severe bleeding the power to kill in a matter of minutes.

1. Open the mouth and remove false teeth or any natural ones that have been knocked out.
2. Taking care to avoid being bitten, explore the back of the mouth and throat with a finger. Remove any solid matter such as vomited food and wipe out with a rag or swab any liquid that has accumulated. Note its nature—blood, food, watery liquid or phlegm. These may occur in various combinations.
3. If other injuries permit, turn the patient onto his side so that the mouth faces downwards and any liquid will run out freely. In case the neck has been damaged the head must be turned carefully at the same time as the rest of the body and supported on a pad so as to keep the neck in line with the rest of the back.

    The limbs should be arranged to steady the injured person, taking care in the movement and disposition of any that have been injured. At least two persons are necessary to turn the patient and when more are available the most reliable of them should be given charge of the injured parts.
4. If the whole patient cannot be turned, turn the head carefully to one side, remembering that the neck may have been injured (*Figure 8.8*), and raise the shoulder on the opposite side on a pad. If the patient is on a stretcher, the foot should be raised a few inches. It is usually recommended that the position of the head should depend on whether the face is pale or congested. Lowering the head is stated to increase the risk of cerebral compression, especially if the face be congested. In fact, congestion may be caused by constriction of the neck by clothing or because

breathing is obstructed. In any case, the practical danger of obstructed breathing outweighs the more theoretical danger of aggravating compression of the brain and a clear air passage helps to reduce the risk of congestive bleeding within the skull.

When the patient must lie supine the jaw must be held forward. This can be done by the method shown in *Figure 8.10*, or with the thumb in the mouth, which is less tiring but may not be applicable if the jaw has been broken.

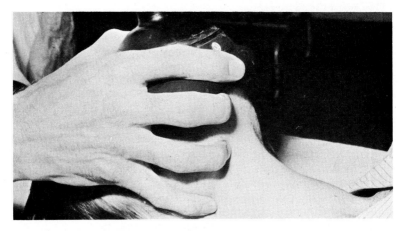

Figure 8.10. Illustration showing the grip that holds the jaw forward. The little finger is placed behind and above the angle of the jaw and must exert considerable pressure. It is not enough to keep the mouth shut

5. If the head cannot be turned to one side because the neck has been injured, the jaw must be held forward and the back of the mouth and throat explored from time to time and cleared out as indicated.

The care of the air passages must be continuous. If two people are available one should be given charge of the head end and suitably instructed while the other deals with other matters. If the First Aider is on his own he must first clear the air passage. If the patient is already lying in a favourable position this should not be disturbed, otherwise the head should be turned to one side; the disadvantages referred to on page 172 should, however, be borne in mind. If there are other injuries to attend to the First Aider must not allow them to claim his whole attention but must assure himself repeatedly and frequently that the patient is still breathing easily.

6. If breathing ceases, clear the air passage and then carry out artificial ventilation.

A conscious patient can look after his own air passage as a rule but should he vomit, which is not unusual, he may need help in clearing his mouth and throat.

Vomiting is a special danger of the unconscious state and may occur at any time, silently and effortlessly. Repeated exploration of the mouth and throat is therefore essential, whatever the position of the patient.

The details of the care of the air passages are of vital importance; obstructed breathing is one of the most urgent and dangerous developments. The proper attitude is to presume it is present in every patient unconscious from whatever cause and to take steps to deal with it. If there has to be a choice between clearing the air passage and arresting serious bleeding the air passage should be given priority because it can usually be cleared very quickly and once cleared it is likely to remain clear while the bleeding is dealt with, which may take longer and require the whole attention of the First Aider.

The management of wounds of the head

A clean dry dressing and nothing else whatever should be applied to wounds of the head; some medicaments, sulphonamides among them, can cause convulsions if they reach the brain.

Bleeding from the scalp may be profuse. Pressure over the occipital or the temporal artery is worth trying but may not slow the bleeding. Direct pressure on a firm pad over the wound is permissible only if there is no doubt at all that the skull is intact. The ring pad has its uses if local pressure cannot be applied but it may be better kept in place by hand than by a bandage. A useful temporary measure is to apply a constrictive bandage just above the eyebrows and ears and to tighten it until the bleeding stops. As with any constrictive bandage, if applied firmly it is likely to cause further bleeding and if applied tightly enough to stop the bleeding it will soon become dangerous. It should be used, and then only for a few minutes at a time, if nothing else staunches the bleeding.

As with bleeding anywhere else, the part should be raised as far as circumstances permit.

It is usually recommended that dressing should be applied lightly over a bleeding ear. Provided that the ear concerned is kept downwards to let the blood run out it does not matter a great deal if no dressing is applied, unless the patient is going to take a long time to reach skilled care.

Blood from the nose or ears should be examined for the watery appearance that indicates escape of cerebrospinal fluid.

MAXILLOFACIAL INJURIES

Maxillofacial injuries have many of the features of craniocerebral injuries and the two are often combined. Because there is damage to the nasal passages and their offshoots as well as to the mouth there is a common risk of obstructed breathing. This is because of bleeding into the nose and mouth and also collapse of the tongue and other soft tissues that have been deprived of the support of their rigid skeleton.

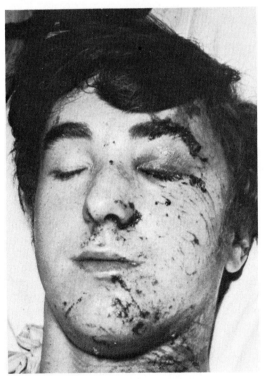

Figure 8.11. The fact that the left cheek bone has been depressed is masked by the swelling of the cheek, but the combination of overlying grazes, black eye and bleeding from the left nostril point clearly to the existence of the fracture

The face is more or less bruised and bloated and the eyes may be closed. The nose may be flattened or displaced and it usually bleeds freely with or without leakage of cerebrospinal fluid. The teeth may be broken and out of line and bloody saliva runs from the mouth. If the patient is conscious he is likely to find speaking and swallowing difficult or impossible.

In the severe cases there is no question of whether the patient should go to hospital but in the milder injuries, especially those restricted to the zygomatic (cheek) bone, it is easy to overlook the presence of a fracture. The signs that should arouse suspicion are bruising and abrasion of the cheek, bleeding from one nostril, double vision, eyes at different levels, numbness or tingling of the cheek, lip and gum and difficulty in opening the mouth. Although the bony support may have been badly dented, swelling of the soft tissues can mask the depression so that there is little or no visible flattening (*Figure 8.11*).

If these injuries are dealt with at once treatment is usually easy, but within a few days the fractures may set quite firmly and be difficult to re-place. Untreated, they can cause ugly deformity and interfere with chewing and ocular movements.

Treatment

Unconsciousness and the air passages should be treated as already described. Because bleeding is often profuse and because the soft parts can cause obstruction the semi-prone position is of especial value whenever it can safely be adopted.

When the jaw is painful, the traditional bandage can be used provided that there is little or no bleeding and the air passage is clear but no attempt should be made to apply it when there is much bleeding because it may then cause or aggravate respiratory obstruction. It is fair to say that to omit the bandage is never serious whereas to apply it can be disastrous. If the patient vomits it must be removed at once. It is useless with a dislocated jaw, which is already locked and consequently self-supporting.

SUMMARY OF FIRST AID

The First Aider has more scope for dramatically successful treatment in the care of the unconscious than with almost any other consequence of accident yet the majority seem to regard an open fracture of a large bone as being more important than unconsciousness.

The air passages

For the purpose of competitions the signs of obstructed breathing can be simulated quite well but the dramatic return of a pink colour to the lips when genuine obstruction has been relieved cannot be reproduced when the lips have been daubed with blue pigment. The details of diagnosis and treatment have to be taught by the spoken and the written word and make less impact on the mind and memory than the physical acts of applying splints and dressings. The following rules should be learned by heart, as with poisons, and applied to every unconscious person, whatever the cause of unconsciousness.

1. Clear the air passages of solid and liquid matter.
2. If possible, turn the whole patient.
3. At least turn the head and, if possible, have it a little lower than the rest of the body.
4. Carry out artificial ventilation if spontaneous breathing fails.

If the patient is breathing quietly and easily

If his lips are pink and free from froth

} his breathing is not obstructed and other conditions urgently in need of treatment should be dealt with.

If the patient is breathing noisily and with difficulty

If his lips are blue

If his lips bear froth

If his chest is sucked in when he inspires

} respiration is obstructed and demands immediate attention.

Breathing that has been obstructed may become so again; repeated examination is essential and further clearing may be required. If the patient remains blue when quiet, easy breathing has been restored:

Look for damage to the chest and treat appropriately.
Oxygen may be used if available.
Oxygen must not be used if the air passage is still obstructed.

Wounds

Apply a clean dressing.

Bleeding may be difficult to control: direct pressure, ring pad, pressure points, a temporary constrictive bandage and raising the head—each has a place in treatment.

The face and jaws

The air passages take priority.

Splinting by bandage is rarely necessary and may aggravate obstructed breathing.

Unconsciousness

There is no First Aid for the unconscious state as such, only for its complications.

Confusion, stupor and coma are unimportant diagnostic labels compared with the ability to recognize that the level of consciousness has changed. The deeply unconscious patient is unresponsive to all stimuli; the normal patient responds normally; confusion and stupor cover the range of responsiveness between.

The local signs may be helpful if accurately observed and reported to the doctor; the patient's general condition is an even more important subject for observation and report.

9

INJURIES OF THE CHEST AND ABDOMEN

Most of the teaching and practice concerning injuries of the limbs and head is based upon experience of these injuries in peacetime conditions. In the case of the chest and abdomen, however, injuries in peacetime are much less frequent than those affecting the limbs and much of the accumulated knowledge is derived from the wounds and injuries of war. These are for the most part obvious and in bygone years were usually fatal. First Aid was largely restricted to dressing wounds and arranging prompt medical care for those who were still alive and little attention needed to be paid to these matters in manuals for civilians.

There are, however, increasing numbers of serious injuries of the trunk in peacetime. Road accidents can lead to crushing or impact affecting the trunk of passengers in vehicles, riders of cycles and pedestrians alike. At present there is much building and the men concerned are liable to fall from heights, be struck or crushed by massive beams, by machinery, vehicles or falls of earth. Advances in medical care have meant that many of these accidents need not be fatal if prompt action can be taken to recognize and, when possible, to treat the immediate effects of injury.

THE CHEST

Structure and function

The chest and its contents are often likened to bellows, driven by the muscles of respiration and causing air to pass in and out of the lungs. As an analogy this is apt to only a very small extent, but the structure and function of the chest and its contents are essentially simple.

Air has to pass freely in and out of the lungs. Its purpose is fulfilled within the air sacs (alveoli) of the lungs, where gases are exchanged between the blood flowing through the lungs and the air ebbing and flowing within the lungs.

Effectual respiration includes the act of breathing and the associated movements of blood and gases. Id depends upon the following:

The muscles of respiration.
Stability of the chest wall.
The ability of the lungs to expand and contract under the influence of the muscles of respiration.
Free passage of air between the atmosphere and the alveoli.
Free passage of blood through the lungs.

Anything that interferes with any of these events can have serious consequences that multiply and extend beyond the chest and the act of respiration. In addition, the heart may suffer directly or indirectly.

THE EFFECTS OF INJURY

Simple fractures

Present manuals of First Aid have little to say about injuries other than fractures of the ribs. These are not infrequent, they are usually restricted to one or two ribs and they are more often uncomfortable than serious

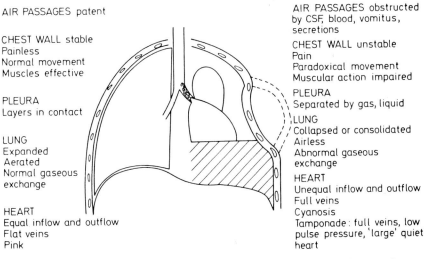

AIR PASSAGES patent

CHEST WALL stable
Painless
Normal movement
Muscles effective

PLEURA
Layers in contact

LUNG
Expanded
Aerated
Normal gaseous
exchange

HEART
Equal inflow and outflow
Flat veins
Pink

AIR PASSAGES obstructed
by CSF, blood, vomitus,
secretions

CHEST WALL unstable
Pain
Paradoxical movement
Muscular action impaired

PLEURA
Separated by gas, liquid

LUNG
Collapsed or consolidated
Airless
Abnormal gaseous
exchange

HEART
Unequal inflow and outflow
Full veins
Cyanosis
Tamponade: full veins, low
pulse pressure, 'large' quiet
heart

Figure 9.1. A composite diagram illustrating the important conditions for normal breathing on the left side of the figure and the various results of injury on the right.
(From London, P. S. (1959). *The Practitioner* **182**, 437)

except in old people and those with diseased lungs. For such persons, the fact that the pain of broken ribs inhibits effectual ventilation and coughing can be very dangerous. Firm support by bandages applied after the patient has breathed out may ease pain but it does little or nothing to maintain effectual ventilation because its comforting effect depends upon restricting movement to the painless range. There is, in fact, little to be gained by applying the standard First Aid for simple fracture of ribs, even as a preliminary to medical care. Medical care should always be arranged because at any stage complications may be detectable only with the aid of radiographs and in the elderly there is serious risk that pneumonia will follow quite mild injuries, simply because they are painful enough to hamper breathing or coughing.

Major injuries

These and their effects are indicated diagrammatically in *Figure 9.1*.

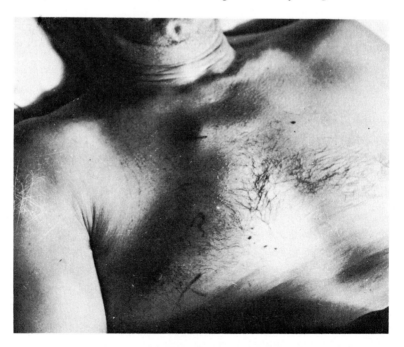

Figure 9.2. Stove-in-chest with obvious subsidence of right 2nd, 3rd and 4th ribs
(From London, P. S. (1959). *The Practitioner* **182**, 437)

The chest wall

Violent impact can break ribs in one or more places each and seriously interfere with respiration. The injured area moves under the influence of changes in air pressure instead of muscular contraction. Normally, when the patient breathes in, the pressure within the chest wall falls and air flows in through the proper channels. If part of the chest wall has lost its stability it will sink in (*Figure 9.2*) as the internal pressure falls and this subsidence occurs at the expense of some of the normal inflow of air. When the patient breathes out the opposite occurs. The unstable part is blown out by the rising pressure within the chest and this occurs at the expense of some of the normal outflow of air.

This movement of part of the chest wall in the opposite direction to normal is known as paradoxical movement and it can have very serious consequences. In mild cases there may be no more interference

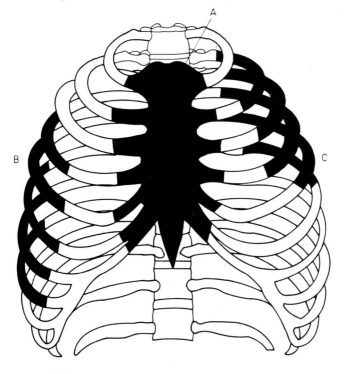

Figure 9.3. Patterns of staving in: (A) anterior, (B) lateral, (C) sub-scapular, often due to a fall on the shoulder. The scapula may also be broken

with breathing than that caused by pain. The affected area may be small or splinted by the weight of the shoulder girdle. In severe cases, when many ribs are broken on one or both sides of the chest (*Figure 9.3*) the effects are striking and grave.

Paradoxical movement reduces ventilation and causes deeper breathing in an attempt to increase the exchange of air between lungs and atmosphere. The effort to breathe more deeply is painful and also unsuccessful because the more vigorous respiratory efforts cause more violent paradoxical movements and set the mediastinum swinging from side to side. Air no longer moves smoothly in and out of the lungs; more and more oxygen is abstracted and more and more carbon dioxide is added with the result that the blood passing through the lungs derives less and less benefit from its passage. The final and fatal stage of this process is a state of equilibrium between the gases in the alveoli and the gases in the blood.

Apart from the paradoxical movement, which may be easily visible in the naked chest and often palpable through clothing, the patient shows:

Cyanosis.
Irregular respiration, usually in the form of short breaths limited by pain. If coughing occurs it is cut short by pain and attempts to speak are similarly hampered.
Sweating.
Anxious expression.
Restlessness that may amount to violent and aggressive activity.

It should be emphasized that paradoxical movement is not always obvious or easily recognized by the inexperienced eye; what is at least as important a sign is the respiratory distress that should not go undetected. When distress is present it needs to be relieved; if paradoxical movement can be detected it merely adds certainty and precision in diagnosis.

The restlessness and unco-operative behaviour and incoherent manner are easily attributed to any known or suspected injury of the head so that the true cause goes unrecognized and untreated. The likelihood of such oversight will be reduced if it is remembered that the restlessness of head injury is not aggressive unless the patient is disturbed, whereas the victim of hypoxia caused by injury of the chest is aggressive without provocation.

The pleura

Normally the layers of the pleura line the chest wall and cover the lung with but a thin film of liquid between them. They are not more easily parted than two plates of metal with a film of oil between them. The layers slide easily upon each other but can be separated only if the seal is broken. Upon this seal depends the lungs' ability to comply with the movements of the chest wall.

Broken ribs cause tearing of the pleura and the intercostal tissues; they may also puncture the lung. Bleeding from the chest wall and leakage of air from the lung break the seal and the lung collapses more or less, according to the amount of blood or air or both around it. The lung loses some of its ability as an organ of gaseous exchange.

An important sign that the lung has been punctured or the trachea or a bronchus torn is subcutaneous emphysema. This is first recognizable as a fine crackling felt under the skin and most often at the site of a broken rib. It may at first be mistaken for bony crepitus, but it often spreads as more air enters the subcutaneous tissues and occasionally causes massive and extensive swelling. If the source of the air is a main air passage, surgical emphysema first becomes evident at the root of the neck.

In spite of the alarmingly inflated appearance that it can cause surgical emphysema as such is not dangerous. It is, however, a danger sign, showing that damage has been done within the chest.

The lungs

Apart from becoming collapsed as described above the lungs may be torn by the broken ends of ribs and the lacerated areas will be surrounded, as in any other tissue, by zones in which blood is effused from its vessels; later this blood evokes inflammatory changes that add to the outflow of liquids into the tissues. These are the changes of consolidation and they can occur without the irruption of broken ribs. Especially with the flexible chest of the young, a blow on the rib cage can injure the lung without causing fracture; the ribs yield at their joints with the spine behind and at the costal cartilages in front. To see the violent paradoxical movements of the intact chest wall of a young person struggling against an obstructed air passage is to gain a vivid appreciation of the flexibility of what is regarded as a fairly rigid structure. Bruising shows on the surface of the lung as bands stamped upon it by the superjacent ribs. It extends deeply and as it does so gradually fades out and becomes diffuse.

Similar changes occur as a result of the violent shock wave of an explosion and were seen during the war (blast lung). The change is simply a widespread and not necessarily uniform effusion of blood into the connective tissues of the lungs and into the air sacs. It can also result from sudden widespread crushing. The extravasation may occur well beyond the lungs, causing suffusion of the skin of the upper part of the chest, the shoulders, face, neck and conjunctivae. This is the picture of traumatic asphyxia. The extravasation may thicken the normally tenuous and readily permeable alveolar layer between blood and air and also may fill the alveoli, but the usual cause is a maldistribution of blood so that instead of going to normally ventilated alveoli it bypasses them or it may supply unventilated alveoli.

The result is a serious interference with the normally easy passage of gases to and from the blood in the capillaries next to the alveoli. In addition, the vessels in the lung may be pressed upon by the effused blood and subsequent inflammatory exudate; they may also undergo constriction caused either by damage or by a reflex. Furthermore, reduced oxygenation and accumulated carbon dioxide can increase the permeability of the tiny vessels and so increase the outflow of liquid from them. These local changes in the lung can so impair oxygenation of the blood as to lead to depression of cerebral function. Consciousness becomes clouded or wholly lost and changes in the brainstem can cause pulmonary oedema.

There is thus a sequence of events that can become not only self-perpetuating but self-aggravating and unless effectually dealt with it can end in death. Such changes can occur very soon after injury without the chest's being affected by the injury, which underlines the necessity for First Aiders to recognize respiratory distress whenever it occurs and do their best to relieve this by whatever means they have, irrespective of the cause. Apart from these changes affecting the chest and its contents there may be the consequences of injury elsewhere, especially bleeding with oligaemic shock and anaemic hypoxia.

The air passages

These may be obstructed rapidly by free bleeding from the lung or from injuries of the face, jaws and pharynx; by cerebrospinal fluid escaping from a fracture of the base of the skull; by vomitus and, rarely, by rupture of a large bronchus. They may be obstructed more slowly by less severe bleeding, by the out-pouring of liquid that characterizes pulmonary oedema and by failure to expel the bronchial secretions. Even with uninjured and previously healthy lungs suppression of coughing will lead within a day or two to wet lungs and then to pneumonia. This was a frequent cause of death during prolonged unconsciousness before the great importance of careful bronchial toilet was recognized. With diseased lungs, abnormal amounts of bronchial secretion increase the urgency of the need to keep the air passages clear. This applies whether coughing is abolished by unconsciousness or suppressed by pain.

The heart

The impact that can damage the lungs may also injure the heart. It may suffer mild and local bruising that does not impair its action or it may suffer severe bruising that can mimic a serious coronary occlusion and lead to shock or congestive heart failure. If the patient survives the initial injury, the bruised muscle may later soften and give way, causing rapid death. The heart or its vessels is sometimes torn and the blood shed is pent within the tough fibrous pericardium. As it accumulates it presses increasingly upon the heart and the clinical picture of cardiac tamponade appears. This is:

1. Weak pulse because of low pulse pressure.
2. Slowing of the pulse during inspiration and speeding during expiration. This is the reverse of the normal changes and is accordingly called pulsus paradoxus.
3. Faint or imperceptible heart beat.
4. Distension of the veins in the neck.

If these signs are present, their meaning is clear but an exsanguinated patient may not show them even when cardiac tamponade has occurred. The First Aider can only do his best in such a difficult and confusing situation; only a doctor can be expected to recognize and treat cardiac tamponade.

The aorta

Another rare but serious effect of injury of the chest is rupture of the aorta, usually where the ligamentum arteriosum connects it to the pulmonary artery. This is usually followed quickly by the death of the victim but if the escaping blood is confined by the surrounding tissues a false aneurysm will develop and may not only escape detection but be compatible with an active life. Suggestive features include unequal force of the radial pulses and distension of the jugular veins. Radiographs show broadening of the shadow cast by the mediastinum. First Aid can do no more than make the patient comfortable until he is in the care of a doctor.

The trachea and bronchus

These structures can also be torn, partly or right across. Rupture of a bronchus may easily escape diagnosis but the rare injury of rupture

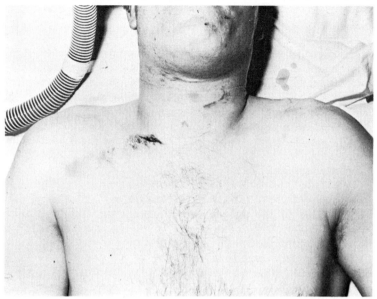

Figure 9.4. Pattern bruising as well as grazes and bruises caused by impact on the throat; the larynx was broken

of the trachea should be suspected when there is a combination of surgical emphysema with pattern bruising of the neck (*Figure 9.4*).

Open injuries

Open injuries vary from small stab and penetrating wounds to extensive destruction, as by shot-gun injuries, and broadly speaking they pose different problems.

Penetrating injuries owe their importance to the fact that the heart, main vessels, air passages, gullet, diaphragm and abdominal viscera may be punctured. At first there may be little or nothing to suggest that serious damage has been done and a tiny breach in the skin may not arouse suspicion of deep and dangerous penetration if the patient appears to be well. The decision that these injuries are not serious can be taken in safety only if the patient has the benefit of detailed observation and investigation in hospital. Signs of shock and bleeding, cardiac failure or tamponade, surgical emphysema, coughing or vomiting of blood, and pain on swallowing are danger signs.

Large wounds of the chest wall carry all the dangers enumerated above together with the liability to infection of any wound. They have in addition a special danger—open pneumothorax. This has many features in common with paradoxical respiration because when there is a large hole into the pleura the lung collapses and the normal pressure changes within the chest are seriously disturbed. The larger the hole, the greater the proportion of air that enters the chest through it instead of through the normal channels; with very large holes the injured person dies promptly from asphyxia. With his dying breaths the patient draws all the air through the hole into the pleural space and none into the lungs. Fatal anoxia develops very rapidly. Severe rupture of the trachea, a main bronchus or the lung also cause open pneumothorax.

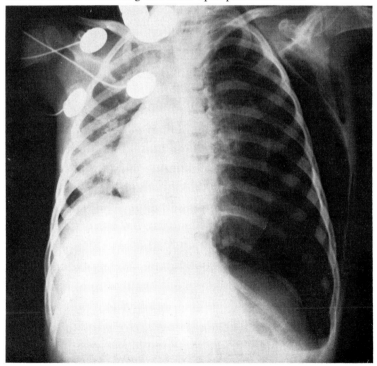

Figure 9.5. Marked collapse of the left lung and displacement of the heart to the right caused by a large pneumothorax

Small holes cause a special pneumothorax because they sometimes open only during inspiration and close during expiration. Air is drawn into the pleural space with each breath but none is expelled. More and more accumulates, the intrapleural pressure rises steadily, squeezes the lung, pushes the mediastinum to the other side and compresses the heart and great vessels (*Figure 9.5*). This condition of so-called tension (more accurately, compressing) pneumothorax leads to increasing respiratory distress, cyanosis, shock and heart failure and is extremely dangerous. The valvular opening may be in the chest wall or in the lung or a large air passage.

Another complication of a torn lung is air embolism but this is beyond treatment either by First Aid or by the full facilities of an expert in thoracic surgery. Fortunately it is rare.

Clinical features of injuries of the chest

The important signs to look for and note in injuries of the chest are:

Obstructed breathing.
Respiratory distress, that is, a struggle to breathe, not necessarily because of obstruction.
Coughing up blood or bloody froth.
Cyanosis.
Discolouration of the skin of the chest, shoulders and face with suffusion of the conjunctivae (traumatic asphyxia).
Distension of the veins in the neck.
Asymmetry of the chest wall, which may be the result of subsidence caused by fracture or collapse of the lung; fullness caused by surgical emphysema, or, less often, compressing pneumothorax. Both can cause crackling under the skin.
Asymmetrical movement of the chest wall, possibly caused by fracture (which inhibits movement or causes paradoxical movement), collapsed lung or pneumothorax.
Shock.

A condition that is sometimes seen is overbreathing tetany. It causes great alarm but is harmless. The characteristic course of events is started by some sort of shock or fright that may be unaccompanied by injury. The victim complains of difficulty in breathing and becomes greatly agitated. The agitation spreads to those around him and is increased when the victim complains of feeling faint and of funny feelings (tingling or pins and needles). He may go on to gasp out that he is losing the use of his hands. By this time alarm and consternation are general and the patient is rushed to medical aid.

The patient is regarded as gasping desperately for breath but a few moments' observation makes it clear that far from having difficulty in getting his breath the patient is in fact breathing both deeply and rapidly.

The condition is of an hysterical nature. There may at first be a feeling of suffocation that causes the patient to take deep breaths; as deep breathing continues the normal residue of carbon dioxide in the lungs and blood is greatly reduced. The blood becomes slightly more alkaline than normal and this causes the tingling and the feeling of weakness or helplessness. The hands may show a characteristic arrangement with the hollow of the palm increased, the fingers nearly straight and extending around the curve of the palm and the thumb drawn across the palm with its tip near the tips of the fingers.

Sometimes the patient can be cajoled or bullied, even shocked by a brisk smack or a douche of cold water, into restraining his breathing or, better still, holding his breath. Failing this, breathing in and out of a bag may enable the concentration of carbon dioxide in the lungs and blood to rise to normal and so relieve the symptoms.

Once seen, the condition is immediately recognizable but on first encounter it can be an alarming experience that may add one more to the agitated retinue. It occurs in both sexes but more often in the young than the mature.

The physical signs of the various types of injury of the chest may seem formidably numerous and complicated but the really important ones—obstructed or distressed breathing, deformity and paradoxical movement, open pneumothorax and cyanosis—are not difficult to remember and are usually readily recognized. Unfortunately they are difficult to simulate.

Severe injuries are not frequent against the background of injuries in general but they deserve careful attention because of the serious results that can develop rapidly and also because First Aid has a big part to play in their management.

Treatment

Obstructed breathing

Much that has been said about this in the chapter on head injuries applies equally to injuries of the chest and it is particularly important to remember that unconsciousness may be accompanied by signs of injury of the head but caused by the hypoxia of obstructed breathing, severe injury of the chest or exsanguination.

Obstructed breathing must be recognized and dealt with promptly but because the cause of the obstruction is often in the lungs it is less easy to deal with than when it arises at the top of the respiratory tract. Bleeding may be both free and continuous and a helpless or unconscious person should therefore be arranged to allow liquids to run out through the mouth. If an hour or more is likely to elapse before medical aid will be available the patient should be turned from one side to the other every hour or so. This helps to prevent liquids from accumulating in the lower of the two lungs. If one side has to be chosen for the patient to lie on it should be the injured one so that if any blood or other liquid should run down the trachea it will go to the damaged rather than the undamaged lung. Another reason is that lying on the injured side will splint it and so help to reduce pain. Unfortunately, the recumbent position is often badly tolerated by those with injured chests and circumstances may make it inadvisable or impossible to change the patient's position. Whenever possible the patient's own efforts to cough and clear his lungs should be assisted and provided that he can do this the position that he finds most comfortable should be allowed; it will often be sitting up.

In the past tracheostomy was occasionally carried out (traditionally with a penknife) as a desperate measure in case of severe respiratory obstruction. For the patient who is far from full surgical facilities it may well be worth while if the doctor has suitable instruments. Though it plays a very important part in the definitive treatment of some injuries of the chest it is less likely to succeed as an emergency measure than the hopeful enthusiast may choose to believe. Methods of tracheal or cricothyroid puncture have been devised with the aid of suitably designed trocar and cannula. They are least likely to be satisfactory in more or less unskilled hands, for which some have been designed, and they may not be a very satisfactory alternative to tracheostomy by a doctor. This is not to suggest that tracheostomy sets should be regarded as a natural part of doctors' First Aid kits; like any appliances, they should as far as possible be used only by those with the knowledge and skill to do so successfully.

Paradoxical movement

When breathing is distressed and whether or not it seems obstructed paradoxical movement should be sought. It is most likely to be found after crushing of the chest, particularly in the case of the driver of a crashed vehicle. It may not be practicable to expose the chest but serious paradoxical movement can be felt through thin layers of clothing. The dangerous consequences arise because of the abnormal movement and the treatment is simply to stop it. It is done most easily by pressing on the unstable segment. This recommendation is directly contrary to the standard First Aid practice, which is intended to avoid damaging the lung. In fact, the damage that the lung has already suffered will not be materially increased if pressure be applied correctly.

Before applying pressure, however, the air passages must be cleared. In some cases this will itself abolish paradoxical movement and it will then be necessary only to guard against its recurrence. If pressure is necessary it should be applied with the hand with just enough force to stop the abnormal movement. This may cause alarming subsidence of the unstable area but the sign of success is easing of the patient's breathing and he may even express his thanks. As an alternative to manual pressure a firm pad of suitable size can be laid on the unstable segment and kept in place by a firm, broad bandage or by making the patient lie on it. If these measures afford no relief they should be abandoned.

A more difficult procedure is to apply mouth-to-mouth breathing in time with the patient's own efforts. It is unlikely to be tolerated by the conscious person but may occasionally be feasible with the unconscious. The manual methods of artificial ventilation can be applied safely to the injured chest. Special care is necessary to clear the air passage and to keep it clear.

As long as paradoxical movement is mild, without distressed breathing, it should be observed but not treated.

Open pneumothorax

When there is an obvious hole in the chest wall the most urgent need is to ventilate the lung that the inrush of air has allowed to collapse. Even a conscious patient may accept mouth-to-mouth ventilation in such a case. Artificial ventilation will get rid of the air that is already in the pleural space and it will also stop the useless flow of air in and out of the hole. It is less urgent to try to seal the hole. A good thick dressing kept firmly in place by one or more broad bandages may prove to be air-tight but it is better to use adhesive tape, if available, and cover the dressing completely with it. Nevertheless, even a dry dressing will at least reduce the flow of air and is therefore better than nothing and once it is moistened by blood it may even become air-tight.

For the First Aider a compressing pneumothorax is something to be suspected rather than treated. Air can be heard being sucked into the chest but there will be no sound of it escaping during expiration. The hole should be sealed as above. For the doctor, however, decompression should be considered. The reasons for decompression are respiratory distress, cyanosis and congested veins in the neck in the patient who has been sucking air into his chest. A wide-bore needle should be inserted into the front of the chest below the clavicle. When the pleura has been entered air will be heard to hiss out. When the hissing has ceased the needle should be removed. The small puncture seals itself.

Because it may not be easy to distinguish between air hissing out and air hissing in unless water-sealed drainage is available, it is important to be sure that a compressing pneumothorax exists before plunging a needle into the chest; otherwise it will induce a pneumothorax and in that event the hissing noise would be made by air passing into the pleural space. This difficulty can be overcome by tying a finger of a rubber glove over the butt of the needle and cutting off the tip; this allows air to pass only outwards. Alternatively, the needle can be mounted on a syringe without its plunger but containing a small amount of sterile water or saline solution to show which way the air is moving.

Cyanosis

Cyanosis is usually caused by defective oxygenation of the blood and the cause may be: obstructed air passages; abnormal movements of the chest wall and lungs; damage to the lung which impedes the exchange of gases between blood and alveoli; impaired action of the heart; or simply depressed respiration resulting from pain or from damage to the brain. Toxic cyanosis need not be considered in this instance.

The important distinction for the First Aider is between cyanosis from obstruction and cyanosis from other causes. The importance of this distinction is all the greater now that ambulances and rescue teams carry oxygen apparatus: Blue lips are not a reason for giving oxygen without further ado. When the patient is cyanotic the following steps should be taken:

1. Make sure the air passage is clear.
2. Deal with an open pneumothorax, if present.
3. Look for paradoxical respiration and stop it if present.
4. Confirm that the air passage is clear.

If the patient is still blue, oxygen should be given. If the patient's colour does not improve with oxygen:

5. Make sure that the apparatus is working properly.
6. Make sure that the mask fits.
7. Review steps 1 and 4.

There is no point in giving oxygen if the mechanics of respiration are at fault nor if it fails to relieve cyanosis.

The question is asked whether 5 per cent carbon dioxide in oxygen is better than pure oxygen. A person in need of oxygen usually has excess carbon dioxide in his lungs and his blood already. Adding to it will not stimulate the respiratory centre because this is already depressed by the excessive carbon dioxide and needs oxygen to revive it.

Two further points about cyanosis need attention. First, if it is mild it is easily overlooked even by the experienced, and if the light is poor or the patient is dirty, marked cyanosis may pass unnoticed. Secondly, the severely shocked patient may be incapable of developing cyanosis. For it to occur, about one-third of the normal quantity of haemoglobin has to be of the reduced kind and sometimes pre-existing anaemia or severe current bleeding may deplete the circulating haemoglobin below the critical level.

The subject of cyanosis has been considered at some length because there is a good deal of confusion about it and it is all too often regarded as a sign that oxygen should be given. Cyanosis is a serious sign and one to be looked for in any unconscious person and any victim of chest injury. It is much more often a sign that breathing is obstructed than that oxygen should be given. Like the tourniquet, oxygen may at times be life-saving, but it is used wrongly more often than not. It is harmless only if the air passages are clear and even then this should be confirmed frequently.

The fact that cyanosis is definitely absent is not to be taken as reassuring if the patient is severely shocked; the air passages and the chest wall should receive attention when necessary.

SUMMARY OF FIRST AID

The treatment of severe injuries of the chest is directed to restoring the effectiveness of the chest as a bellows, of the lungs as organs of gaseous exchange and of the trachea and bronchi as conduits. For the surgical team in a hospital this may mean tracheostomy, bronchial toilet, providing artificial ventilation or perhaps stabilizing the chest wall, aspirating blood and air from the pleural space, relieving cardiac tamponade and resuscitating by blood transfusion, all within a short time of receiving the injured person (*Figure 9.6*). Against this elaborate background the First Aider may feel helpless but, properly trained, he

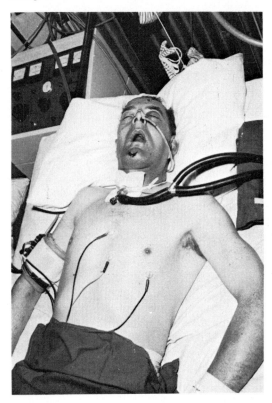

Figure 9.6. Nasal feeding, tracheostomy, artificial ventilation and continuous recording of electrocardiogram, blood pressure and pulse rate in the treatment of a stove-in chest. There were also fractures in the lower limb

may be able to do much to keep the patient alive until he can reach skilled help and his observations may be of great value to the doctor; indeed there are conditions in which the eyes and the hands can be more reliable and more accurate than radiographs and, unlike radiographs, they are available to all and they can be applied as soon as the patient is seen.

1. Clear the air passages by posture or coughing.
2. Seal any sucking holes in the chest wall.
3. Arrest severe paradoxical movement by pressure on the unstable segment, by hand, by pad or by lying the patient on that side.

These measures are urgently required and must take precedence over everything except very severe bleeding.

4. Give oxygen only if cyanosis persists after these measures have been carried out.
5. Any puncture wound of the chest wall is to be regarded as dangerous, especially if there is surgical emphysema around it.
6. Relieve pain and distress. A conscious patient may adopt the most comfortable position, usually sitting up. A broad bandage firmly applied may be comforting. It should not be used unless it is.

Danger signs other than those mentioned above include:

1. Spreading surgical emphysema without a wound.
2. Increasing respiratory distress, especially if the chest wall is undamaged and the air passages are clear.
3. Coughing of froth or blood.
4. Distension of the veins in the neck even when the head is raised.
5. Widespread purple staining of the upper part of the body with blood beneath the conjunctivae (traumatic asphyxia).
6. Increasing shock.

For these, First Aid has nothing to offer except prompt movement to medical care and a report of what has happened.

THE ABDOMEN

Wounds of the abdominal wall

Wounds of the abdominal wall must all be regarded as serious, however small, whatever the patient's condition and however confident he may be that penetration was very slight. Apart from gunshot and deliberate stabbing, wounds may be inflicted by falls on sharp objects and by accidental knife wounds. A butcher's knife may slip when a joint is being boned and can perforate the bowel in several places. With small wounds the bowel may seal itself and not leak for several hours. During this time the victim may seem perfectly well.

Apart from wounds of what the laymen accepts as his belly, it must be remembered that wounds of the lower part of the chest, the flanks, loins and buttocks may penetrate abdominal organs. A fall in the sitting position may cause broomsticks, chair-legs and the like to enter the anus or vulva and penetrate deeply among the entrails. There may be little or no bruising and little or no bleeding from the natural orifices of the perineum but the fact that a fall of this kind has occurred demands prompt medical care. A fall astride a bar or ridge may rupture the urethra. Bruising in the perineum and blood exuding from the penis are danger signs. The skin is usually not breached.

The standard teaching about posture, dressing and the care of protruding gut needs no comment. It is a remarkable fact, however, that spontaneous rupture of abdominal scars and escape of bowel is not a shocking procedure. People have walked to hospital with their guts in their trousers and in one instance an elderly woman spent the weekend in bed with her bowels because she did not wish to trouble her doctor! Her consideration was happily rewarded by her uneventful recovery after operation.

Closed injuries of the abdomen

It has long been known that trivial and even unperceived blows upon the abdominal wall can rupture the spleen, liver, kidneys, bowel and even the pancreas. It is perhaps less well known that severe injuries of this nature can occur without causing any pain or sense of malaise for periods that vary from several hours to several days.

Once there is knowledge or even suspicion that the abdomen may have been struck or crushed, the following signs are important:

Pain or nausea.
Vomiting.
Signs of shock.
Marks or tenderness upon the abdomen (including flanks and loins).
Brown or red discoloration of the urine.

If the person concerned is otherwise uninjured, it should be made clear to him that if he declines to see a doctor it is upon his own responsibility. The First Aider's responsibility ceases when he has warned against the possible consequences of neglect.

When other injuries make it inevitable that the patient will go to a doctor, the First Aider has little to offer in the treatment of closed injuries of the abdomen. His main duties are to recognize that injuries may have occurred, to forbid anything to eat or drink and to preserve, if possible, any specimen of vomitus, urine or faeces. None of these should, of course, be deliberately sought.

Apart from cases in which the abdomen is known to have been injured, suspicion of internal damage should be aroused by:

1. Vomiting, whether bloody or not, when it is accompanied or followed by abdominal pain. Bloody vomitus is less important if there has been any bleeding from the mouth or nose.
2. Blood in the urine or from the bowel.
3. Spreading or worsening pain in the belly.
4. Collapse of shock without obvious cause.

It should be emphasized that head injuries do not cause clinical shock; if the picture of shock occurs in the unconscious person without other injury sufficient to explain it, the abdomen should be suspected.

Important as these signs are, they are not quite as certain in their meaning as a sign that may be described as pattern bruising, which is the pattern of clothing imprinted on the skin as a bruise. For this to happen, the skin must be supported by an unyielding surface when the blow is struck. When the skin is immediately supported in this way, as it is on the shin, pattern bruising has no serious significance, but when such a bruise is seen on the yielding part of the abdominal wall it means that this has been crushed against the spine or the pelvis and that the interposed muscles and viscera have been damaged and must be explored. In an unconscious patient with other severe injuries pattern bruising of the anterior abdominal wall may be the only sign of potentially fatal internal injury.

Whether they are open or closed, certain or suspected, abdominal injuries brook no delay. Bowel may begin to leak or severe bleeding occur at any time. In the early stages treatment is usually a simple surgical procedure but if treatment is delayed the surgeon may find peritonitis instead of an easily sutured perforation; he may have a gravely exsanguinated person urgently in need of an operation to staunch the bleeding; in short, he has the complications and not just the injury to deal with. With these injuries there is no place for hopeful expectancy or self-medication.

10

INJURIES OF THE PELVIS AND SPINE

THE PELVIS

Types of fracture

There are two main types of fracture, the mild and the severe.

Mild fractures

These affect the processes and the rami of the pubis (*Figure 10.1*). Fractures of the processes do not often occur. They are usually caused by avulsion forces and occur mainly in young and vigorously athletic people whose muscles are strong enough to pull off one or other of the anterior spines of the ilium or the tuberosity of the ischium before these growing parts have undergone bony fusion by obliteration of the epiphyseal cartilage.

They should be suspected when there is a history of violent muscular effort followed by pain in the region of either the groin or the buttock. The painful area is swollen and tender; in the groin, bruising may appear within an hour or so as a faint bluish discoloration, but in the buttock it may appear only after a day or two and perhaps some distance away. Active movements of the hip are painful but the patient. may be able to hobble with assistance.

Definitive treatment is a matter of making the injured person comfortable while helping him to start moving the limb as soon as possible. For First Aid, a comfortable position is all that is required; bandages, splints and compresses are unnecessary.

The the layman pain and swelling in the groin after effort may mean 'rupture'. For the First Aider the distinction between mild fracture and rupture is unnecessary because both require medical treatment.

Fractures of the pubic rami are more often found in older persons and usually follow a fall or a stumble, sometimes direct violence. The painful swelling near the groin and the painful movement of the hip may be indistinguishable from fracture of the neck of the femur without

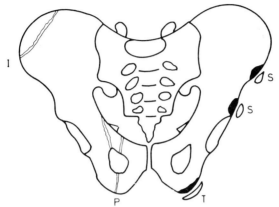

Figure 10.1. Mild fractures of the pelvis. I: crack in ilium. P: fissures in pubic area. SS: avulsed iliac spines. T: avulsed tuberosity of ischium

X-ray examination. The facts that there is no shortening of the limb and that it is not rolled outwards on its side do not rule out a fracture of the neck of the femur. The patient should be made comfortable with the legs supported. They need not be splinted but the pain may be eased by tying the legs together with pads between them. The pelvis does not need to be supported by a broad sling or bandage and should other conditions make it desirable the patient may be sat up or laid on one side.

These fractures produce little or no shock as a rule.

Severe fractures (*Figure 10.2*)

Great violence is responsible and the usual causes are falls from a height, forcible crushing and the violent impact of road accidents on passengers or pedestrians. The injuring force may be applied to much of the body to cause other severe injuries, notable among which is rupture of the diaphragm.

The broken bones of the pelvis are widely displaced and disrupt extensively the adjoining cellular tissues. Widespread bleeding occurs from other small vessels and sometimes from large arteries as well.

Shock is consequently severe and may come on rapidly, especially in old persons because they tolerate bleeding less well than the young with their more adaptable circulations.

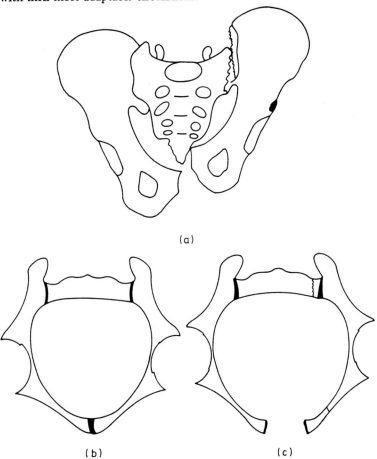

(a)

(b)   (c)

Figure 10.2. Severe fractures. (a) Disruption of symphysis, fracture near sacro-iliac joint and displacement of the innominate bone. The urethra may be torn. (b) Cross-section of normal pelvis viewed from above. (c) 'Book' pelvis. The symphysis has been widely separated (and may tear the urethra) and fracture has occurred in the sacro-iliac region. Other fractures may also occur

In spite of the dramatic nature of the accident and the severe damage caused, these injuries can be overlooked when there are others or when there is unconsciousness or severe shock. The patient may be in no state to feel pain and his complaints may not be about the pelvis.

In thin people swelling may be obvious and palpation of the ridges and spines of the pelvis may reveal asymmetry, abnormal mobility and crepitus. In fat people, on the other hand, swelling may be masked and it may be impossible to recognize either deformity or instability of the pelvis but the patient cannot walk and any movement of the trunk or legs is likely to be painful. Blood tracks up the abdominal wall and there may be complaints of abdominal pain with tenderness; there is often swelling between the navel and the pubes.

Apart from these effects, severe fractures of the pelvis are sometimes complicated by damage to the urethra and, less often, to the bladder. The urethra of the female is almost immune because it is short and not closely related and tethered to the pubic arch as it is in the male. The urethra is torn either as part of the general disruption of the soft tissues that accompanies displacement of the bony framework or because a fragment of bone has injured it directly. For the First Aider it is an injury to be suspected rather than diagnosed confidently. There is often a little blood at the urinary meatus of the penis, sometimes frank bleeding. Whether this be present or not the patient should be allowed to pass urine if he feels like doing so. He is, however, unlikely to do this unless a long time has elapsed since injury and enabled the bladder to become uncomfortably full. The matter is therefore most likely to require consideration where hospitals are few and communications poor. For a doctor it would in such circumstances be permissible to attempt to relieve the distended bladder by passing a catheter or, failing this, by suprapubic puncture with a suitable needle. Suprapubic cystostomy should not be used because it might handicap early surgical repair and allow infection to enter the pelvic haematoma. The reversal of the previous warning against passing urine has been made for two reasons. Firstly, if the urethra has been torn the patient is unlikely to be able to pass his water, but, secondly, should he do so, the escape of sterile urine into the tissues is not serious. Fear of infection used to be the reason for the warning. Passing a catheter is now regarded less favourably than it was because it has been suggested that many ruptures of the urethra are incomplete so that passing a catheter may complete the tear and complicate recovery whereas if closed suprapubic drainage is used without even attempting to pass a urethral catheter the urethra remains in continuity and it is later possible to pass a suitable instrument and show that there is a way past the site of injury and into the bladder without need to repair the rupture.

Some severe fractures make the pelvis resemble a book placed on its spine; the sides sag apart under the influence of gravity aided by the natural tendency of the limbs to roll outwards (*Figures 10.2b* and *c*). It may therefore be comforting to the patient to have a firm supporting bandage or binder passed round the pelvis and the legs and feet bound together.

These injuries require urgent treatment because there is usually severe internal bleeding and it may be necessary to operate to repair internal injuries. Given favourable circumstances, the results of prompt treatment can be very gratifying and the classical disasters of extravasation of urine, infection, stricture and fistulae after rupture of the urethra can be entirely avoided.

Perhaps the most important single step in First Aid is gentle handling and conveyance of the patient. Any movement is likely to affect the broken pelvis and aggravate shock.

Another type of injury to the urethra may conveniently be considered here although it is not associated with fracture. It is caused by a violent upward blow on the perineum such as may occur when a person falls astride a bar or ridge. Again, it is only the male urethra that is vulnerable in this way by being crushed against the pubic arch. There is likely to be blood at the external urinary meatus; swelling and bruising soon appear in the perineum from where they spread into the root of the penis. Early operation is required to repair this type of rupture of the urethra.

Rare complications are injuries of the great vessels and nerves that run close to the bone. Unless there is external bleeding, however, First Aid can only try to expedite medical attention.

Fracture-dislocation of the hip

A dislocated hip is characterized by a fixed deformity in which the thigh is flexed, adducted and medially rotated. A fracture-dislocation is less obvious because the back of the acetabulum has been broken off. With a simple dislocation the head of the femur is jammed behind the intact rim of the acetabulum but when this has been broken off the head of the femur is not fixed. The limb may lie in a natural position and unless the patient complains of the area the very existence of the injury can be overlooked. An unconscious and restless patient may divert suspicion by moving the limb, and another reason for overlooking the injury of the hip is that there is a fracture of the same thigh. The First Aider can be excused this error although he may justifiably be warned that the combination occurs (*Figure 10.3*). There is, however, swelling and tenderness in the area and a sentient patient may complain of numbness, tingling or paralysis of the limb. The sciatic nerve runs close to the acetabulum and is not infrequently injured by a fracture-dislocation (*Figure 5.13*). Another form of fracture-dislocation

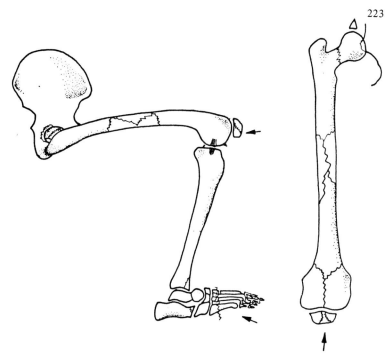

Figure 10.3. Characteristic patterns of injury in the lower limb of motor drivers and passengers. Note the combination of injuries that can occur

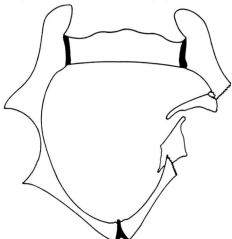

Figure 10.4. Inward fracture-dislocation of hip or stove-in pelvis

occurs when the head of the femur is driven so hard into the acetabulum as to break it and pass some way into the pelvis (*Figure 10.4*).
The signs are as described above but occasionally the pelvic organs
are damaged.

It is sufficient to support the legs comfortably and bind them
together. Shock may be severe after this injury.

THE BACK AND SPINE

First Aid is required for a number of conditions other than fractures
and dislocations. The serious injuries carry the special risk of damage
to the spinal cord and nerves but because many different results of
injury have painful disability in common it is necessary to cast the net
of diagnosis more widely than in the manuals of First Aid.

The significance of symptoms and signs of spinal disorder

Clinical experience and experiment have shown clearly that pain in
the region of the spine and in the limbs and trunk can be produced by irritating the soft tissues both around and within the vertebral
column. The capsules and ligaments of joints, the periosteum, the
muscles and the dura mater are all sensitive to pain, which may be felt
locally or at a distance. It is debated whether bone itself is sensitive
but there are sufficient other sources of pain to make it irrelevant
whether bone is sensitive or not. This means that many different
injuries and diseases of the spine cause similar groups of signs and
symptoms and they do this because they affect the soft tissues in the
same way, by squeezing them or stretching them. A spinal abscess
squeezes by its bulk and stretches because it is enlarging; a spinal tumour
has the same effects. A sprain stretches; a displaced intervertebral
disc can stretch or squeeze or both. A dislocation or a fracture does
not simply stretch; it rends violently and the displaced or distorted
bone then presses.

Weakness or paralysis, numbness, tingling or a feeling of deadness
are evidence that the spinal cord or nerves are under pressure, stretched
or torn.

It follows from this that it may be difficult to distinguish between
serious and mild injuries and between injuries and diseases. The presence
or absence of a recognized injury is not a reliable criterion because a
supposed injury may bring to light a disease whereas the apparently
causeless onset of severe disablement may mean nothing more serious

than that a familiar action has caught the spine, as it were, off guard.

If there are signs of damage to the spinal cord or nerves the patient must evidently be handled with great care but even if these signs are absent it is not always safe to assume that there is no cause for anxiety nor any need for care.

Sprains

As a diagnostic term, sprain is rarely applied to spinal disorders. A sprained neck is usually diagnosed as traumatic torticollis or wry neck and a lumbar sprain as lumbago, 'rheumatism' or 'fibrositis'. In many cases there has been no incident that could be regarded as an injury. A draught, damp or cold is blamed because it is not widely understood what great forces act on the spinal structures during everyday activities such as turning one's head or reaching forward for a small object. In the ordinary way the forces concerned are largely absorbed by the correctly co-ordinated activity of the spinal muscles and the sensitive ligaments of the spine are protected from strain. If there is any inco-ordination of muscular activity or if the joints are worn by age and so more difficult to control accurately, abnormal forces may act momentarily upon vulnerable and sensitive structures.

Everyone is familiar with a sprained ankle. There is a well recognized moment of injury, the pain is localized, swelling can be seen and tenderness found in the painful place. In the case of a sprained spinal joint, however, the lesion is deeply seated, there may be no recognized injury, there is no swelling, tenderness is diffuse and not directly over the spine. Pain is also not localized and may be felt far away from the spine. The striking differences between the two conditions seemingly demand different diagnostic terms and even different types of lesion.

The work of Lewis and Kellgren among others has done much to show that the differences are more apparent than real. Irritation of the deep tissues of the spine can produce signs and symptoms a considerable distance away. Lesions of the cervical, thoracic or lumbar spine can cause pain respectively in the head, arm, trunk or lower limb. Much of the credit won by osteopaths and less reputable manipulators has come from their ability to relieve such pains, especially when they have been ascribed to disorders of the viscera and never connected with the spine.

The sprained spine is painful to move, the affected part may be held in a position of deformity and there is usually tenderness in the area. Pain may be felt to radiate from the spinal region or may occur apparently entirely separate from it. There is neither swelling nor bruising nor clearly defined tenderness over the vertebrae.

226

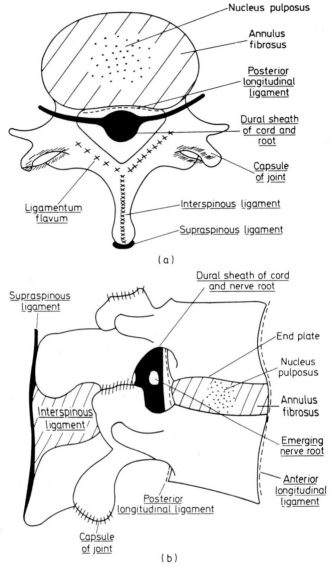

Figure 10.5. The intervertebral disc and related structures. Those underlined have been shown to be sensitive and to cause lumbago and sciatica when suitably stimulated. The closely packed muscles in this area have been omitted. (a) Diagrammatic top view of a vertebra and disc. (b) Side view

Lumbago and sciatica

Lumbago and sciatica are terms of respectable antiquity but they have lost some of their former popularity since the intervertebral disc came to be blamed for much painful disability. They are, however, useful terms provided that they are recognized as denoting symptoms and not specific diseases, and they have the advantage of not being associated in the lay mind with persistent disability. Lumbago is acute and sometimes crippling pain in the back; sciatica is pain felt down the limb in the course of the sciatic nerve and its branches. These symptoms are usually ascribed to 'disc lesions' or 'slipped disc' but have other causes, which include sprains.

The intervertebral discs (*Figure 10.5*) separate the bodies of the individual vertebrae and comprise a blob of soft matter, the nucleus

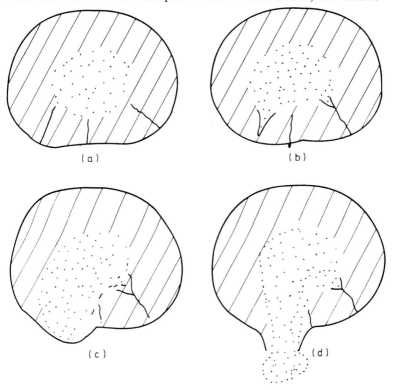

Figure 10.6. Diagram of intervertebral disc showing the progress of events from mere cracking to frank extrusion of nuclear material. This may occur in any direction but causes symptoms only when it goes backwards (c and d)

pulposus, enclosed within a ring of tough fibrous tissue, the annulus fibrosus. Above and below, the nucleus pulposus is bounded by the bony surfaces of the vertebral bodies. Often referred to as shock absorbers they are better regarded as allowing the spine to bend by providing flexible bonds between the vertebrae. The intervertebral discs develop degenerative changes in early adult life and among other effects of degeneration the annulus fibrosus loses its normal elasticity and develops cracks (*Figure 10.6a*). The malleable nucleus pulposus may be forced into these cracks, widening them and causing the thinned annulus to bulge and perhaps give way so that the nucleus itself irrupts into the spinal canal. According to whether the prominence is in the midline or to one side it approaches the coverings of either the spinal cord or its nerve roots and if large enough it can squeeze the cord itself or its nerves (*Figures 10.6b, c, d; 10.5a*).

Protrusion may occur suddenly either as a result of movement that is recognized as being injurious, or for no evident reason. It is not necessary to lift a heavy weight—an apparently innocuous action may suffice—and if attack follows attack the exciting cause often becomes progressively less obvious. In these cases it is likely that protrusion is aggravated or recurs from time to time; there may be almost continuous discomfort in the back or there may be long periods without any symptoms whatever. For all the popularity of the term 'slipped disc', discs do not slip; they may be extruded, they may prolapse or they may protrude.

When there is no pressure upon the spinal cord or its nerves the signs and symptoms are much the same as for sprains. When the cord or nerves are pressed on the patient complains of numbness and tingling or that the limb feels dead or heavy or that it is clumsy and weak. The pain may be continuous and severe or the patient may be fairly comfortable at rest but suffer severe stabbing or shooting pain in the back or leg if he moves or coughs. Complete paralysis, even of a single muscle or group of muscles, is exceptional but weakness may be found, most often in the extensor of the great toe. Disturbed action of the bladder is a rare but serious sign that requires careful attention (*see* page 221).

All that First Aid can provide is comfort and this often means merely assisting the sufferer to get into the position that he finds most comfortable and avoiding any disturbance thereafter. In such a case there is no objection to analgesic drugs such as aspirin or codeine or to putting a suitably protected hot-water bottle on the painful area. Should the patient become unconscious the bottle must be removed at once.

Fractures and dislocations

Fractures and dislocations fall into two main groups, the mild and the serious. Except with pathological fractures there is always an unmistakable injury. The spine is one of the most frequent sites of pathological fracture because it is especially liable both to secondary tumours and to weakening by osteoporosis in the aged. When the cause is osteoporosis a pathological fracture is of little importance; when fracture is caused by malignant disease the patient is unlikely to survive for long.

Mild fractures

These are the result of either pulling (*Figure 10.7a*) or crushing (*Figure 10.7b*). The usual sites for traction fractures are in the lumbar transverse processes and the lowest spinous process of the neck. The transverse processes are sometimes broken by a heavy, localized blow, but usually by violent twisting or bending of the spine. They are deeply buried and though very painful they cause only rather diffuse tenderness in the loin. The lumbar fascia is very strong and may prevent bruising or swelling from appearing at the surface.

The spinous process of the 7th cervical vertebra is pulled off when a vigorous movement of the arms and shoulders is stopped dead. Unless

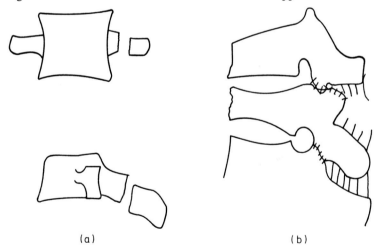

(a)   (b)

Figure 10.7(a). Avulsion fractures of transverse and spinous processes. (b) Crush fracture of body

the muscles of the shoulder relax instantaneously they can pull off this most prominent and isolated point of attachment. Pain, tenderness, swelling and bruising develop quickly and are precisely over the avulsed bone, which may be movable under the fingers.

Crush injuries follow falls, and whether the person concerned lands on his feet, his buttocks, his shoulders or his head the spine is forcibly flexed and one or more vertebral bodies may be crushed. The injury may affect only the bone but in many cases the ligaments behind are stretched or torn. There is, therefore, usually some tenderness, swelling and bruising over the spinous processes of the broken vertebrae.

With these injuries the spinal cord and nerves are in no danger but occasionally forced flexion of the thoracic spine causes the sternum to bend and snap and organs in the chest can be damaged.

Serious fractures

These are often accompanied by dislocation, and it is this that damages the spinal cord and is therefore the more serious feature. They are caused by great violence and most often affect the lower part of the neck and the junction of the thoracic and lumbar parts of the spine. The damage to the spine is usually done by crushing, flexing and twisting forces. Extension is rarely responsible for serious injuries of the vertebral column but it can damage the spinal cord even though there be neither fracture nor dislocation and the only sign of such an injury (*Figure 8.8*) may be a mark of damage on the face or brow.

Serious fractures and fracture-dislocations are most often caused by falls, road accidents or falls of roof in mines. The patient does not usually appear shocked unless there are other injuries. Indeed, there is a rather striking tranquility about many of the victims of severe spinal injury. They feel as if they have been cut in two and lost the body beyond the injury. There is pain at the site of injury and if the back is disturbed it shoots round the body or into the limbs even though they are paralysed.

When first seen the injured person may be spread-eagled and unable to move. He may indeed be dead. If the neck has been injured the head is often held askew and any attempt to move it will be resisted by a conscious patient. If the cord has escaped injury the victim of a broken neck may be found with his head in his hands and unwilling to let go. He may, however, be able to walk about unaided and consequently attract little attention, especially if several persons have been injured (*Figure 6.1*). In this instance the patient complained only that his neck was stiff after he had dived into shallow water.

The signs of spinal injury are pain and tenderness at the injured place and there is usually also swelling and a definite gap where the ligaments have been torn between the spinous processes (*Figure 10.7b*). Gaps and swelling are less easily recognized in the neck than lower down because in the neck the spinous processes are deeply embedded in the tough ligamentum nuchae whereas lower down there is only a thin supraspinous ligament. Whenever possible the back of any seriously injured person should be examined. It is not always desirable to expose the back but if a hand is run down the spine irregularities of contour and consistency may be found. For First Aid purposes they are to be regarded as certain evidence of severe injury and such signs can be more informative than radiographs.

Injuries of the spinal cord

Being surrounded by the bony rings of the vertebrae the spinal cord will be endangered if the rings become displaced. Generally speaking, the

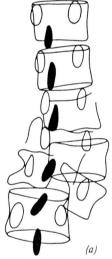

(a)

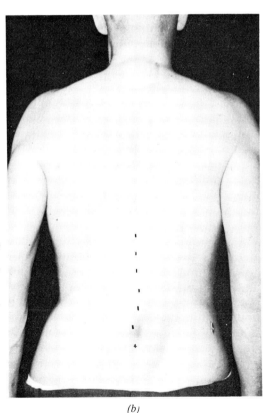

Figure 10.8. In spite of the severe deformity shown by the tracing of a radiograph (a) there was little external evidence of it (b), and there was no more than slight damage to one or two nerve roots. Note that the spinous processes, which have been picked out with black, show little deviation from a straight line

(b)

greater the displacement the more severe the damage to the cord but startling displacement can occur and yet the cord escape (*Figure 10.8*). On the other hand, the cord can be irreparably damaged without there being any damage to the bones.

In old persons the intervertebral discs of the neck bulge and may ossify to form hard transverse ridges projecting as much as 5 or 6 mm backwards towards the cord. This most often occurs between the 5th and 6th cervical vertebrae, at which level the cord is swollen by the large numbers of nerve cells that supply the arms. This leaves less room than at other levels and sudden violent movements of the head and neck can cause the cord to be crushed against these ridges. When the movement is one of extension the spinal canal can be further encroached upon by inward bulging of the ligamenta flava behind (*Figure 10.9*). All

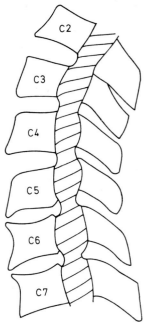

Figure 10.9. Diagrammatic longitudinal section through the neck when bent well back. The vertebral canal is encroached upon from in front by hard ridges, which are largest between C5, 6 and 7. The encroachment from behind by ligamenta flava ceases when the neck is straight or bent forward

degrees of injury from mild and wholly recoverable bruising to complete destruction of the spinal cord can occur and there may be none of the signs of injury to the vertebral column and its ligaments.

Spinal paralysis

This may be partial or complete. Paralysis of the legs is known as paraplegia and of all four limbs as tetraplegia. The damage does not necessarily affect the cord evenly throughout its thickness and because the paths of movement and feeling do not run together there is sometimes paralysis on one side and loss of feeling mainly on the other side (*Figure 10.10*).

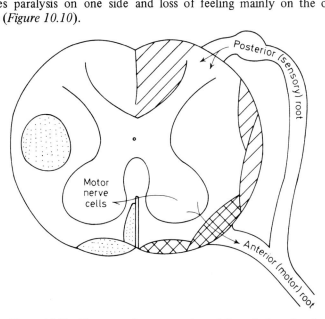

Figure 10.10. Diagrammatic cross section of the spinal cord and nerve roots. The dotted areas represent tracts of fibres controlling movement; close dots are for tracts that change sides on the way from brain to muscle; sparse dots for those that do not. Striped areas are for tracts carrying sensation and not changing sides. Cross-hatched tracts carry sensation and change sides. All these and other tracts occupy both sides of the cord and mingle closely. Nerve roots also occur on each side. They convey the nerve fibres of which the parent cells lie in the spinal cord. The cells are connected by the various tracts to different parts of the brain

When it first comes on paralysis leaves the affected muscles completely limp. The legs are usually paralysed throughout and remain in any position but when the arms are affected paralysis is rarely complete and the active muscles impose characteristic positions on the limbs. When the injury is at the level of the 5th and 6th cervical vertebrae the arms may lie beside the head; when the damage is a segment lower they are by the sides with the forearms resting on the trunk.

If the cord has been crushed it cannot recover. First Aid, and surgery for that matter, are incapable of bringing about recovery but careful handling may prevent partial paralysis from becoming complete. This is of especial importance with injuries at the thoracolumbar junction because here the spinal canal is occupied by both the cord and its nerve roots (*Figure 10.11*). Unlike the cord, injured nerve roots may be able to recover so that a person who is at first paralysed in both legs may

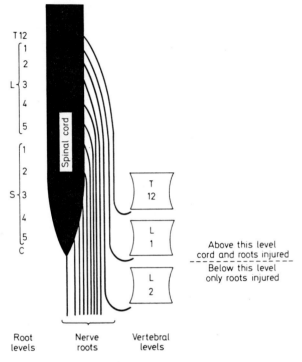

Figure 10.11. Diagram showing how the level of injury determines whether spinal roots are affected alone or with the cord

regain the use of them because their nerves recover; control of the bladder, which rests in the cord, is permanently lost. Only by careful handling can any chance of recovery be preserved.

Paralysis apart from the limbs

When the spinal cord has been crushed or severed, movement and feeling are lost in all organs and tissues supplied from below the level of injury of tracts or nerves. When the lowest part of the spine has been injured only nerves are affected and paralysis is confined to the legs. Above the junction of the thoracic and lumbar regions of the vertebral column the spinal cord may also suffer. Its lowest segments control the bowel and bladder. The immediate result is that the bladder relaxes but its sphincters close. Urine accumulates but because the bladder has been deprived of feeling the paralysed person is unaware that it is full. It may be much distended and easily felt, or seen in a thin person, as a rounded swelling rising from behind the pubis. Fortunately the bladder empties itself eventually because the pressure within can overcome the closed sphincters. First Aid need not therefore concern itself with emptying the bladder but if this occurs automatically the clothing should be carefully removed and the patient dried. The bowels usually remain confined for several days and can therefore be ignored at first.

Injuries in the upper reaches of the spinal cord deprive the abdominal viscera of their nerve supply. The abdominal wall is usually slack and painless at first but it often becomes distended after a while because the bowels are paralysed and gradually become blown up by digestive juices and gas collecting within them. There is still no pain and if serious abdominal injury has occurred as well it easily goes unrecognized (*see below*).

Another important effect of injuries high in the spinal cord is to abolish sweating and vasomotor control. The sympathetic nerve fibres that control these functions leave the cord between the first thoracic and the first or second lumbar segments, which means that if the cord is crushed in the neck the person concerned has in effect undergone total sympathectomy. The blood pressure may be well below normal but the pulse pressure is not much reduced and the force of the pulse is usually reassuring. The skin is on the pale side, but warm and dry because sweating has been abolished, and the patient is alert. This satisfactory state can easily be seriously disturbed because the loss of vasomotor control renders the patient liable to postural fainting. For this reason, if circumstances make it impossible to keep a paraplegic or tetraplegic person's body horizontal, it is safer for him to be tilted head down than head up.

The combination of spinal and other injuries

In the unconscious patient the fact that spinal injury has occurred may easily escape consideration and more often than not it is not recognized. Signs that should arouse suspicion of spinal injury include: bruise, graze or other injury on the face or forehead; unexpected dryness of the skin of the lower part of the body; complete limpness and lack of spontaneous or reactive movement in two or four limbs; no reaction to disturbance of obviously injured limbs; and a see-saw alteration of movement of the chest and belly during breathing. If there is any reason to suspect that spinal injury has occurred, the patient must be treated with due care; any necessary extension of the neck must be carried out cautiously when there is a possibility that it has been broken.

The victim of paraplegia or tetraplegia without other injuries does not usually show signs of serious shock after the immediate effects of the injury have passed off, but with the loss of feeling and vasomotor control in much of the body special care is necessary to avoid over-looking serious associated injuries.

Moderate pallor and a warm, dry skin are to be expected; a conscious patient is usually tranquil and clear in his mind. Suspicion of other injuries should be aroused should the skin become paler, the pulse rate rise and its force lessen. Clouding of the mind or mental distress are strong hints that serious bleeding has occurred and if no source is evident the trunk should be suspected.

These facts are important because spinal injury on its own is not in urgent need of skilled care. Delay should certainly be avoided but if there has to be a choice between, say, severe haemorrhage, large wounds, deepening unconsciousness or serious injury of the chest on the one hand and spinal injury on the other, the spinal case should not be given priority unless complicated by other injuries.

Early dangers to survival after spinal injury

If the cord is not injured above the lowest part of the neck adequate ventilation can be carried out by the diaphragm alone, which makes the belly and chest move in and out in see-saw fashion. As long as there is no cyanosis and breathing is not noisy no treatment is necessary but the patient must be watched carefully because the diaphragm alone is not able to achieve much more than the essential ventilation; any obstruction of the air passages or congestion of the lungs at once endangers survival and must be relieved.

When circumstances prevent the patient from reaching skilled care for a day or two, the bruising and swelling of the spinal cord may spread and cause the level of paralysis and numbness to rise slightly. In most cases this does not affect the chance of survival but when the neck has been broken it may kill the patient. At first the phrenic nerve (arising mainly from the 4th cervical segment of the cord) is unaffected so that the patient can breathe with his diaphragm, but spread of bruising and swelling from segments immediately below this level may cause ventilation to fail. The lips become blue, breathing becomes laboured and secretions accumulate in the throat, where they can be heard rattling with each breath. The condition is distressing to the attendant as well as to the victim. All that can be done is to apply the usual methods of clearing the air passages in the hope that this will succeed but the outcome in such cases is almost always fatal. Mouth-to-mouth ventilation may keep the patient alive for a while and if skilled help can be expected within an hour or so it should be applied, taking care to clear the air passages every few minutes. It must be admitted, however, that such efforts are likely to prove to have been wasted.

THE GENERAL CARE OF INJURIES OF THE BACK

Broadly speaking, pain in the region of the spine that comes on after a wrench or jar from moving a heavy weight is unlikely to be very serious. If the patient can walk he may be allowed to do so, otherwise he should be made comfortable, for which local warmth may help. It is sufficient to get him home and have his doctor see him there.

If pain over the spine radiates down the limbs or around the trunk or if it is accompanied by numbness, weakness or tingling in the limbs, it should be regarded seriously whether there has been an injury or not. Pathological fracture may have occurred (usually after middle age) or part of an intervertebral disc may be pressing on the spinal cord or its emergent roots. The patient should be kept at rest and seen by a doctor without delay.

If pain in the spine comes on after injury by direct violence, crushing, twisting or bending, it should be regarded seriously whether the pain spreads or not and whether or not there is numbness, weakness or tingling elsewhere. If the back can be examined and bruising, tenderness or irregularity of the bony landmarks are found, serious injury is confirmed.

If the patient has lost the use of limbs or bladder special care is necessary.

The management of serious injuries of the back

The main objects in the management of serious injuries of the back are to protect the spinal cord and nerves, to provide comfort and to arrange prompt medical care, in that order.

If the patient is conscious he should be asked about numbness, weakness, paralysis, pain and injuries apart from the back. If he cannot move his limbs they must be examined for injury, remembering that if the cord has been damaged there will be no pain to warn either the patient or his attendant that injury has occurred. Reliance must therefore be placed on looking and feeling carefully for wounds, swelling, irregularity and deformity. Any injuries found or suspected must be treated appropriately. If the back is accessible it should be examined, by both eye and hand if possible, before altering the patient's position. If the patient is on his back already a hand should be passed under him in search of signs of injury, but taking care if there is broken glass about. There is no harm in asking the conscious person if he feels able to move his spine. Should he do so without complaint or difficulty one may be reassured. This appeal to the injured person to test himself can be of great value; he is unlikely to endanger himself but it must be stressed that he should only be asked if he can move. He should not be instructed to move and least of all should he be made to move.

If the patient is shocked or unconscious, special care in examination is required if serious oversights are to be avoided.

Once it has been established that the back has suffered serious injury, with or without damage to the cord and nerves, the patient must be prepared for his journey to hospital.

Handling persons with spinal injuries

The general rule for handling those with fractures of the limbs apply equally to those with fractures of the spine; the broken bones must be prevented as far as possible from moving on each other. This is specially important in the case of the spine, where extra and disastrous damage may be done.

In the conscious patient the injured area is splinted to some extent by the muscles there (*Figure 6.1*) and the patient's ability to complain of pain in the injured area is a further safeguard. If the patient is unconscious even greater care is necessary.

When a victim of accident complains of pain in the back or that he has lost the use of one or more limbs, the neck and back should be examined at once. If the back can be exposed without moving the patient, so much the better, otherwise the examination must be by hand only. The only conditions that must be given precedence are, as in all cases, embarrassed respiration and severe bleeding.

A comfortable position need not be disturbed unless other injuries require it. It does not matter whether the injured person is on his face, his side or his back; all these positions are used in the nursing of paraplegics. Distorted limbs should be straightened carefully after they have been examined for signs of injury, but no attempt should be made to correct deformities of the spine, which should be supported by pads or pillows. If the patient's position has to be altered his spine must be moved in one piece with the head, shoulders and pelvis kept in the same relative positions.

However soon the injured person is expected to reach hospital precautions must always be taken to avoid pressure on insensitive skin because the seeds of pressure sores can be sown within an hour or two of injury. A normal person adjusts his position every few minutes; the movements may be unconscious and very small but they suffice to ease pressure on different areas in turn and to allow blood to flow freely through them once more. Paralysed parts lie like logs; the only movements are carried out by others and unless pressure is widely distributed and frequently relieved where skin, fat and soft tissues can be squeezed against bone they lose their blood supply and can die within a few hours. The following action should be taken by the First Aider:

1. The supporting surface should be firm.
2. Wrinkled and crumpled clothing or blankets must be smoothed out so that the patient lies on a surface that is flat as well as firm.
3. Hard objects such as buckles and badges should be moved from under the patient and bunches of keys or coins removed from pockets.
4. Wherever possible the natural hollows of the body in the position adopted should be filled with firm pads. The head needs support, especially if the patient lies on his side.
5. Bony prominences should be protected from pressure by pads under the calves if the patient is on his back, or between the knees and feet if on his side. Pads should also be placed under the loin or the hip.
6. Constrictions such as garters, straps and shoe laces should be looked for and loosened.

If several hours elapse between injury and arrival in hospital the patient's position should be changed every two hours. He should lie in turn on one side, the back and the other side. The legs should be moved by one person, the shoulders and pelvis by a second and, if the neck has been injured, the head by a third. If there are only two people and the legs have not been injured they should be moved after the trunk. The new position of the patient requires readjustment of pads or pillows. If a leg has been broken it is often better managed without splints, special care being taken over moving and supporting it with pads. If splints are used they must be carefully padded and the un-injured as well as the injured leg must be protected from pressure by splints and knots.

SUMMARY OF FIRST AID

1. Fractures of the pelvis may be so mild as to resemble simple bruises, sprains or strain. If the patient can move either the legs or the trunk it is sufficient to make him comfortable. Splints and bandages are unnecessary.
2. In the conscious patient severe fractures of the pelvis can usually be suspected even if they cannot be diagnosed confidently. In the unconscious or otherwise seriously injured person they can easily be overlooked.

    Support for the pelvis and lower limb is desirable, particularly if the patient has to undergo a long or disturbing journey.

    Internal organs may be injured and the most frequent com-plication is shock caused by severe internal haemorrhage. Careful handling and prompt medical attention are more important than any other measures the First Aider can take.
3. Pain in the neck or back following twists and mild injuries requires a comfortable position. Medical treatment is not urgent.
4. Pain, numbness or tingling affecting the limbs after apparently mild injuries require prompt medical attention. The patient should be put at rest and made comfortable.
5. (*a*) Severe injuries of the spine, with or without loss of feeling or movement, require careful handling and support of the patient lest the damage be aggravated.

    (*b*) Spinal injury alone is not a desperate emergency compared with severe embarrassment of breathing, severe bleeding or deepening unconsciousness.

    (*c*) Spinal injury with paralysis may mask serious injuries in the paralysed part of the body. Obvious clinical shock suggests that hitherto unsuspected injuries have occurred and demands prompt medical attention.
6. There is no one 'best' or 'correct' position for the victim of spinal injury.

7. For short periods, the patient may be left in a comfortably supported posture. Hard surfaces must be padded and hard objects removed from pockets.
8. If several hours will elapse before the patient can receive medical attention, he should be turned carefully every two hours.

11

ORGANIZATION AND SPEED

The purpose of treatment is to further the well-being of the patient as far as circumstances allow. Organization must therefore depend on the prevailing conditions, extracting advantage from good conditions and minimizing the dangers and disadvantages inherent in unfavourable circumstances. Even within the British Isles there is a wide range of conditions, from the short distances and effective services in large towns and cities to the Highlands of Scotland where the nearest ambulance may be 40 or 50 miles away, hospital further still and weather alarmingly unpredictable. In other countries, the distances between medical aid posts of any sort may be enormous, the terrain formidable and the climate extreme.

The organization of medical services has to deal with the number and disposition of staff, equipment and buildings, collection and conveyance of patients, and the emergency movement of medical and supporting staff. The organization of First Aid must fit this pattern and the methods of treatment may vary considerably in different places and at different times.

Broadly speaking, the medical services fall into three groups:

(I)   Full facilities readily available
(II) Full facilities at a distance
(III) Scanty facilities

GROUP I: FULL FACILITIES READILY AVAILABLE

These are the conditions to be found in or near any well developed town or city. Hospitals with facilities for dealing with all grades of emergency cases are close at hand or are readily and quickly reached by an effective ambulance service.

In these conditions First Aid must concentrate on avoiding delay in getting the injured, and especially the seriously injured, to hospital. If this can be achieved within a matter of minutes First Aid will have been adequate if it has merely ensured a clear air passage, arrested severe external bleeding, sealed a sucking wound of the chest, done something to diminish severe paradoxical respiration and avoided further injury or disturbance. In the course of a few minutes' journey exposed wounds are unlikely to become contaminated but if adequate cover (*see* Chapter 3) can be provided without causing delay it should be done. Unless the inflatable sort are available splints are often unnecessary and giving anything to drink is a crime.

With serious emergencies it is popularly believed that the victims are, and should be, 'rushed' to hospital, but those who have been so rushed have been outspoken in their condemnation of unseemly haste. A smooth journey is preferable to one that is merely speedy. Even on the best roads travelling in a modern ambulance can be a nauseating and distressing experience. For the sake of a smooth journey it will often be justifiable to follow a slightly longer route. In built-up areas the co-operation of the police is of great help but the dramatic side of the occasion may need to be played down. The police are only too willing to help and to ensure a clear passage through busy streets; although this is a great advantage they should be politely but firmly instructed that a high-speed journey is not what is required. The following case illustrates this.

A doctor accompanied his injured patient by helicopter and motor ambulance. The flight of some 80 miles was noisy and accommodation was cramped but it did not upset the passengers. The ride of a few miles by ambulance from airport to hospital was made at high speed behind an enthusiastic police escort and it left the doctor badly shaken; his patient was too young and too ill to express a point of view, but recovered.

Destination

It is the understandable wish of the First Aider to consign his patient to the nearest hospital but in fact the nearest hospital may be wholly unsuitable for dealing with the case. Generally speaking the destination of the victim of any particular mishap, whether the result of disease or injury, is laid down by ambulance regulations for the locality. Ambulance crews are usually well aware, however, when this is not a satisfactory arrangement and are justifiably and outspokenly critical of the fact that in some places delays begin only when the patient reaches the hospital.

There may be no medical staff in residence or the doctors may be otherwise engaged when a seriously injured person is brought in.

First Aiders and ambulance crews can do little about this but it is increasingly recognized that the nearest hospital is not necessarily the one best fitted by staff and equipment to deal with the seriously injured. Where there is a choice it is generally better for the casualty to go to the nearest hospital that can be relied upon to meet his needs. In urban areas this is not likely to lengthen the journey much and in any case the time spent by a seriously injured person in a small hospital will be wasted if there are inadequate facilities for treatment and he must still be transferred. As far as possible those responsible for organizing accident services should relieve the First Aider or ambulance driver of any need to decide for himself who should go where but they may be well advised to consult the ambulance service before making rules.

It is at present almost always the case that an injured person for whom an ambulance is summoned will be taken to hospital. This is a wise regulation because although many patients can be looked after adequately at home it is not for the First Aider to try to distinguish between the genuinely and the apparently trivial.

Industrial First Aid

In factories and other more or less self-contained industrial communities there may be good medical services readily available and the First Aiders may then have to decide whether these services should be called upon or whether victims of accident should go straight to hospital. In such circumstances it is the duty of the medical services to provide clear guidance for their First Aid contingents.

In other factories there is no more than a First Aid Box or an 'Ambulance Room' where minor injuries can receive attention. The equipment and staff are governed by regulation and depend upon the number of persons employed. It is unfortunately the case that unless there is careful supervision the facilities actually available often fall far short of what is laid down. Used stock is not replenished, 'sterile' dressings are opened and left open and the equipment may be dirty or defective because of deterioration with age. When there is no more highly trained person available First Aid workers should be prepared to accept some responsibility for seeing that the statutory regulations are complied with. The book dealing with occupational First Aid and published by the St. John Ambulance Association and Brigade is an admirable source of this information.

The relationship of the First Aider with hospitals

It is also worth remembering that the choice between keeping the patient and sending him to hospital does not necessarily have to be made by the First Aider on his own responsibility. In cases of difficulty he should seek guidance over the telephone. This is not often done and it must be admitted that hospitals might not take kindly to it. To some extent this estrangement can be reduced by personal contact with the hospital and some hospitals arrange various forms of demonstration for First Aiders or allow them to spend time in the casualty or equivalent departments. Such contacts are best established at fairly high level so as to minimize the possibility of misunderstanding with the frequently changing casualty officers. First Aiders are sometimes rebuffed by hospital medical staffs and much could be done to foster harmonious relationships if there were good will on both sides.

A useful means of trying to improve relations and communications is to offer the hospital helpful information to which the doctor there makes helpful reply (*Figure 11.1*).

GROUP II: FULL FACILITIES AT A DISTANCE

Full facilities may be available but delay is inevitable because of distance or the nature of the journey. Even in highly developed countries train crashes, mining accidents and mishaps on mountains are followed by delay in treatment that can be reduced but not eliminated by modern means of transport. Aircraft are now much used but their value is limited by weather, terrain and the number of casualties. For all its ability to travel straight up and down and to hover, a helicopter is not always practicable for rescuing casualties from awkward places and there may be no alternative to carriage by hand. In these conditions a more elaborate form of First Aid may be appropriate but how and when it is applied will depend on the circumstances. What would be practicable with room to spare would be impossible in the confined space of a coal mine and at times the injured person cannot be reached for a long time. The First Aider may then be compelled to stand by while rescue teams are clearing debris and gaining access to the patient. If there is nothing else to claim his attention he may at least be able to speak encouragingly to the trapped casualty; he should also be making what preparations he can to apply First Aid when this becomes possible; and if extrication is going to take some time, he may meanwhile be better engaged elsewhere.

Hospital
Registration No. ....

TRANSFER FORM

TO BE COMPLETED AT FACTORY
Items in RED — ESSENTIAL
Items in BLACK — HELPFUL but NOT ESSENTIAL

Date ....

PATIENT	**NEXT OF KIN**	**FAMILY DOCTOR**
Family Name Mr. Mrs. Miss	Relationship	Name ....
Other Names	Name	....
Address	Address	Address ....
....	....	....
....	....	....
Date of Birth	'Phone No.	....
Clock No.	Informed .... Yes/No	....

FACTORY UNIT	**FACTORY RESOURCES:** STAFF		FACILITIES	
Name	Doctor Full Time	☐	Heat Treatment	☐
Address	Doctor Part Time	☐	Tetanus Toxoid	☐
	S.R.N.	☐	X-ray	☐
	S.E.N.	☐	Others—Specify	
	First Aider	☐	....	
Phone No.	Chiropodist	☐	....	
If **transport** available for **patient**	Physiotherapist	☐	....	
'Phone No.	Others—Specify		....	
	....		....	

HOSPITAL TO REPLY TO	**PATIENT'S WORK (Brief Description)**
Name	
Address	

SPACE FOR ADDITIONAL INFORMATION.

THIS PAGE TO BE **DETACHED** AND **RETAINED BY HOSPITAL IN PATIENT'S NOTES**
A 10 SB. C8248

Figure 11.1. A form that supplies useful information to the medical staff who may be unfamiliar with the facilities available at the firm and in turn allows the medical staff to send useful information to the firm

Patient's Name ....

Clock Number ....

TO BE COMPLETED AT FACTORY

HISTORY OF INJURY/ILLNESS

Date................Time................Accident/onset of Illness

Personal History		
Diabetic	☐
Epileptic	☐
Steroids	☐
Anticoagulants ...	☐
Allergic to	

SUSPECTED INJURY/ILLNESS

Tetanus State

Immune	☐
Not Immune	☐
Partially immune ...	☐
Unknown	☐

TREATMENT GIVEN AT FACTORY

Signed by ....
M.O./S.R.N./S.E.N./First Aider.

'Phone No. ....

HOSPITAL REPLY

Registration	Physician/Surgeon	Hospital ....
Date............Time........	Dr./Mr.	Patient's Registration No. ....

EXAMINATION (Please state if b.i.d.)

X-RAY FINDINGS	**DIAGNOSIS**

TREATMENT AT HOSPITAL (including Minor Operation Notes)

Original Copy Signed by ....
M.O./S.R.N./S.E.N.

REQUEST FOR FOLLOW-UP CARE AT FACTORY	**DISPOSAL**	**UNFIT** for work ... ... ☐
	Admitted to	**FIT** for work ... ... ☐
	Ward	**MAY WORK but MUST AVOID**
	Discharged ... ... ☐	(1) Shift work ... ... ☐
	Referred G.P. ... ☐	(2) Any/strenuous effort ... ☐
	Referred Factory ... ☐	(3) Any/continuous standing ... ☐
	NEXT HOSPITAL APPT.	(4) Bending/Lifting ... ... ☐
		(5) Unprotected heights ... ☐
	Date	(6) Food Handling ... ... ☐
	Time	(7) Driving ... ... ☐
	Dept.	(8)

THIS PAGE TO BE RETURNED TO FACTORY WHEN COMPLETED.

As in any other emergency, the first aim must be to save life. Apart from bleeding and obstructed breathing there may be failure of respiration caused by crushing or a noxious atmosphere. If there is danger from fire, explosion or collapse of wreckage all treatment may have to wait until the patient has reached safety.

Firm, secure dressings and comfortable support of broken limbs are of great importance to any injured person who has to be manhandled. For the lower limb Thomas's splint or one of its successful modifications is of great value and may be part of the equipment of a rescue team. Though it may take 20 minutes or more to apply it this time will have been well spent if the casualty is not going to reach hospital for several hours. It is, however, likely to be supplanted by the more compact if less robust inflatable splint. 'Contour splinting' using plaster of Paris is effectual but less convenient than the other methods.

As in Group I, there may be a choice of hospitals. When many hours have elapsed before any treatment has been provided there is much to be said for taking seriously injured persons to the nearest hospital, however small it may be. The victims of severe injury travel badly and may benefit from an opportunity to rest and recover as far as their powers of recovery permit. The time that has elapsed since the accident may have allowed a cottage hospital to send for help in the form of staff and facilities for resuscitation. A First Aider's foresight in the early stages may enable such preparations to be set in motion.

Resuscitation teams

If hospitals are prepared to send out a resuscitation team it may be asked whether this should be summoned to the scene of the accident. The opportunities for resuscitation on the spot may not be good and what can usefully be done at the scene of the accident may be better done in hospital. A resuscitation team would be overwhelmed, or left impotent, by large numbers of casualties whereas in a hospital it would have better opportunities for sorting patients, assessing priorities and acting to the best advantage. In principle, however, there is no doubt that no accident service is complete unless it can supply a doctor or team when called upon to do so by a responsible person. Experience suggests that the need for such an 'outdoor' medical service differs a good deal from place to place and the subject will be considered further in the next chapter.

Morphine is popularly regarded as the most important drug at the scene of an accident and this belief is fostered by newspapers' accounts of how doctors have gone to great lengths to reach casualties and inject morphine. The place of morphine has already been dealt with and leaves the value of these endeavours—often heroic—in question. Were it not for its weight and bulk, Entonox would probably supplant morphine entirely.

Intravenous infusion of blood, plasma or a substitute is outside the province of civil First Aid, but these substances are much in the news and deserve brief consideration.

As the tables in Chapter 2 show, a fair proportion of those dying from injuries do so before they reach hospital and, moreover, they die from haemorrhage. Some lives might be saved by transfusion started at the scene of the accident and the flying squads for obstetric emergencies may seem applicable to other sorts of severe bleeding. The difficulties of starting and maintaining a successful transfusion in the confusion of an emergency can be considerable but resuscitation certainly has a place if a hospital nearby is used to collect and sort the seriously injured. When an injured person can be freed and moved rapidly to hospital this is almost always the best policy but there are undoubtedly a few occasions on which transfusion on the spot is practicable and beneficial. The necessary organization is, however, a part of the organization of accident services in general and not the province of First Aid.

In large-scale accidents First Aiders will soon come under the direction of a police, fire or other officer but where there are only a few casualties the First Aider may have to rely largely on himself and any available help to deal with what confronts him and inform the proper authorities.

Organization of accident services

There is an increasing awareness of the shortcomings of the facilities for treating serious accidents and there is still hope that more will be done to develop, co-ordinate and rationalize what are in many places fragmentary and even chaotic arrangements.

In the hospitals approved for receiving seriously injured persons the outstanding need is for a suitably trained staff to be immediately available. There needs to be a resuscitation unit in which the patient can receive urgent treatment and also be subjected to the sometimes complicated process of diagnosis. The proper working of such a unit depends on having supporting services such as radiography, pathology, blood transfusion and operating theatres promptly available. As well as these facilities on the spot it may be necessary to call in specialists in other fields of surgery or medicine. In Great Britain, where accident services already exist they have usually been associated with orthopaedic surgery but in some countries they are grouped with the emergency cases of surgery and medicine in general, and in others 'traumatology' is an accepted subdivision of surgery. Recent appointments to the staff of hospitals in Great Britain reflect the recognition that casualty, or accident and emergency, departments are having to do some of the work that used to be done by general practitioners and that the doctors in charge need to be skilled in resuscitation and in diagnosis and primary treatment of a wide range of ills and hurts.

Apart from the changes in the hospitals themselves it is likely that suitable hospitals will be expected to provide advice or practical assistance at short notice on a larger scale than hitherto. The working of emergency teams has to be co-ordinated with the duties of police, fire, ambulance and other emergency services; in some parts of the country there is direct radio communication between hospital and ambulance. In the general plan to deal with disasters First Aiders would be of great value, especially as members of organized groups that could be called out. The value of such groups is already well recognized.

This account of the elaborate measures appropriate to an accident service may leave the present day First Aider a little wistful and perhaps envious of the dramatic role of the medical services, but he should be encouraged to regard himself as a valuable part of the service. It is not simply a matter of being assured of this in his training and in special lectures but it means also that the medical and nursing staffs of hospitals should be aware of the place of First Aid as a preliminary to their own activities. They should recognize the enthusiasm and willingness of First Aiders and be urged to spare them at least a few moments to offer a word of encouragement or advice or to elicit information that only the First Aider or ambulance attendant from the scene of the accident may be able to give. This information is at times of great importance.

GROUP III: SCANTY FACILITIES

This group includes large and sparsely populated areas in which the nearest doctor may be a hundred or more miles away and the nearest hospital considerably further. In these conditions everyone should be encouraged to be his own First Aider but this is practicable only where the bulk of the population have a more or less civilized education. Most primitive peoples have their own methods of folk medicine and their own practitioners but the results are not usually comparable with those of orthodox medicine and First Aid.

Even more than in Group II, the more leisurely and elaborate methods of First Aid may be of great value. The Australian Royal Flying Doctor Service and a similar African service, summoned by radio, have reduced the vast distances of those countries to relatively short periods of comfortable travel and the Scottish Highlands and Islands air service has brought similar advantages in Britain. In many parts of the world the injured person must stay where he is or must face the hazards and the rigours of a long journey. As elsewhere, the comfort and smoothness of a journey is more important than its speed. Judicious delay to await a suitable conveyance may be preferable to a prompt start in whatever is available. The most important requirements are a means of raising the alarm and then good communication.

In these conditions many of the severe injuries will be fatal and the urgent life-saving measures appropriate in Group I will often do no more than prolong the casualty's life for a few minutes or hours. For those who survive the immediate effects and early complications of their injuries, eventual recovery is likely to depend on nursing rather than First Aid in the usual sense.

When medical care will be long delayed the chance of recovery may depend upon being able to do something more about bleeding than merely stopping it, if possible. The value of transfusion on the spot in Group II was questioned but in the conditions of Group III it deserves further consideration. A large railway or aircraft accident in a fairly thickly populated country poses entirely different problems from the single individual seriously injured on, say, a farm, plantation or construction project 'out in the bush' or its equivalent. For them, mobile First Aid units might render valuable service while awaiting medical care, and indeed have been set up in a number of different countries.

The armed forces have trained some of their medical orderlies to give intravenous injections and there does not seem to be any strong argument against teaching selected members of mobile First Aid units to do the same. Blood transfusions would not be practicable because of the difficulty of storage and the need for very careful tests to ensure compatibility of the blood of the donor with that of the recipient. There is no substitute for blood, but dried plasma, dextran or even saline will at least increase the volume of blood in circulation and may keep the patient alive while red cells are slowly restored. They have the advantage of not requiring special tests but plasma occasionally causes jaundice and dextran cannot be given safely in amounts exceeding the normal plasma volume (2–3 litres in an adult).

Similar considerations apply to accidents on board ships, where shelter, space and time are available.

Onerous decisions

Broadly speaking, the old saying that while there is life there is hope should guide the First Aider in these difficult and worrying conditions but he should have some idea of what can and what cannot be done to save life. This may be of practical importance if he has to deal with several casualties with injuries of differing severities because by attending to inevitably fatal injuries he may unwittingly allow less serious conditions to deteriorate gravely.

Burns offer the least unreliable guide to outcome. If more than 30 per cent of the body's surface has been burned the prospects of survival without special care are slim; if more than 50 per cent has been burned, the possibility of survival can be dismissed. Apart from liberal drinks and intravenous plasma or dextran there is little that can be done for the patient's general condition. The burns should be wrapped in clean or sterile cloths or, if conditions allow, exposed and allowed to develop dry crusts.

With other injuries that menace life, after trying to ensure a clear air passage and effectual ventilation and to stop accessible bleeding, the First Aider can legitimately revert to some of the old style 'treatment for shock'. There will be no anaesthetic and provided that the patient is not suspected of having suffered abdominal injury, can swallow and does not vomit, he may be allowed drinks as required, in repeated small quantities.

The treatment of wounds in Group III conditions may be carried further than a clean dressing and formal splintage and a cautious attempt to reduce deformity of fractures may be appropriate.

Exposure

The effects of exposure are likely to be met in isolated places in the course of hill walks and mountaineering expeditions where a combination of terrain, weather and lack of assistance means that help is unobtainable for many hours.

The most important fact about exposure is that it can usually be avoided by taking knowledgeable advice about routes, local conditions and clothing. It is most likely to occur when unsuitably clad novices set out into unfamiliar districts where the weather is treacherous. It can also occur when even the most carefully equipped and planned expedition meets unforeseeable difficulties.

The condition depends upon the body's becoming unable to maintain its normal temperature because of, usually, a combination of cold and damp. The first signs are fatigue, failure to keep up with the others, staggering and clouding of the mind, and they require immediate attention. The victim must at once be put and kept at rest because further activity makes matters worse. He should as far as possible be sheltered and warmly wrapped in dry clothing. Warm food or drink is permissible but alcohol is not.

The circumstances will determine whether it is better for the party to shelter together or for some to go in search of help. After rescue, a victim of exposure should be put into a warm bath. No other means of heating is permissible and the chilled parts should not be rubbed in an effort to warm them up.

A similar condition affects old persons living alone when they may be unable to protect themselves against the effects of very cold weather. Exposure and chilling are the cause of many deaths after shipwreck, and can kill unexpectedly quickly in what might be regarded as quite warm waters. If there is warning of disaster it is best

---

ADVICE ON ENTERING THE WATER
(To be broadcast before abandoning ship.)

If you have to enter the water:
1. Put on warm clothing as well as a life-jacket.
2. Once clear of the ship, remain still and float in your life-jacket unless you can see land or a rescue craft close enough to reach by swimming.
3. Do not take alcohol except in small amounts and with sugary food.

In very cold water:
1. Wear gloves and footwear as well as other clothes and a life-jacket.
2. Never try to swim more than a few yards without a life-jacket or other support.

Figure 11.2. The sort of notice that Professor Keatinge would like to see posted on all ships' bridges

to don warm clothing and, if immersed, to keep as still as possible because swimming increases the loss of heat from the body (*Figure 11.2*). Treatment after rescue is as for other sorts of exposure.

Heatstroke

This is almost the opposite of the effect of exposure. It is most likely to occur as a result of exertion in hot damp air, which prevents the cooling effect of evaporating sweat. The early signs are much as with exposure but the skin is very hot and dry. Treatment should start at once, which means that however awkward the place is the patient should not be moved more than a very short distance just for convenience. He should be stripped, fanned and sprinkled with water. Even when ice is available it should not be used because it causes vasoconstriction and so defeats its own object because it prevents evaporation from the skin.

If cooling measures can be continued in transit there is every justification for the earliest possible move to medical care. Drinking is permissible if the patient is conscious.

It can be objected that these are measures far beyond the scope of First Aid as laid down in the manuals, but the need exists for some sort of care for those injured in isolated places and with their widespread influence and long experience of training the unskilled the First Aid organizations seem to be well fitted to help to meet that need. The practical details set out in this book apply for the most part to the conditions prevailing in Britain and comparably developed countries and are not universally applicable. In contrast, the principles of the care of the injured, which have also been set out, are universally applicable and can be used as a basis for First Aid adapted to different conditions or graded in various levels of skill and ability.

12

TRENDS IN FIRST AID AND OTHER EMERGENCY CARE

If the words First Aid are restricted to the subject promoted by the voluntary aid societies it cannot be said that there have been any very striking trends. The joint First Aid manual of the three voluntary societies is now in its third edition and each is notably different from the one before. There is still much that is traditional and of doubtful value but at least unlikely to lead to harm even if it is not likely to have any obviously beneficial effect. Nevertheless, there is a trend away from treatment for treatment's sake and towards a generally more up-to-date and realistic application of current medical knowledge.

This process has been carried a good deal further by authors of books that are independent of the voluntary societies and have not to conform to the uniformity of procedure that is necessary in conditions of competitions as well as genuine operational experience. Dead wood has been cleared away without loss of practical value and interest has been added by explanation and example.

One may justifiably ask, however, what restriction should be put upon the two words 'First' and 'Aid' when used in that order. This question is prompted, among other things, by the frequent use of the expression 'First Aid treatment'. If one goes back to the beginnings of First Aid the two words were used because they precisely connoted what useful first steps could be taken to assist the victims, of injury in particular. The proper emphasis on improvisation makes it reasonable to offer the following definition of First Aid: whatever treatment can usefully be provided by whoever is first on the scene, using whatever is to hand. This at once increases the scope of First Aid to include the most modern methods of diagnosis and treatment such as may be immediately available to a person knocked down in the road outside a comprehensive accident unit. This extension is not unreasonable in the light of the existence of flying squads and special accident and emergency services made up of doctors and ambulancemen with special training and equipment.

Apart from these dramatic and extreme extensions of the concept of First Aid there is the special training given in industry where First Aiders have to face particular hazards of one sort or another. In some factories special techniques of rescue dominate the treatment of the casualty, in others the management of industrial hazards may require skilled medical attention. Occupational First Aid can properly be regarded as a subject in its own right, but with special subdivisions that may differ a good deal from each other.

TRAINING AND ORGANIZATION

Ambulance Aid

Until the report in 1966 of a working party on training in the ambulance service it was of no more than financial advantage to crews to possess a

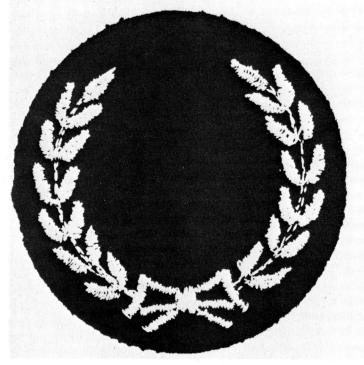

Figure 12.1. Ambulance services' proficiency badge

valid First Aid certificate issued by one of the voluntary aid societies. The working party recognized that great changes had taken place since a report of 1951. Apart from advances in resuscitation in particular and the care of the sick and injured in general, reorganization of hospital services was reducing the number of accident centres and so increasing travelling time during which patients would be dependent upon ambulance crews for their well-being and even their survival. There was also a growing feeling within the ambulance service as a whole that because of the work its members did and the responsibilities they bore they deserved better than being classed as manual workers and merited also a standard of training that was more in keeping with what they had to do.

The working party recommended a course of training for 6 weeks on entry, with a certificate of proficiency (*Figure 12.1*) that was awarded after a year of satisfactory operational service. This recommendation was accepted by the government, together with others dealing with refresher courses.

This training went far beyond what had previously been regarded as First Aid and in order to assist the distinction the term Ambulance Aid was put forward and has been widely accepted. It is, nevertheless, in practice more often that not First Aid in the literal sense referred to.

Advanced First Aid

At the same time, the working party recognized that some ambulancemen would have both the wish and the ability to be trained to higher standards yet and it went as far as suggesting the conditions that should govern the award of an advanced certificate of proficiency. Since then, events have overtaken these suggestions in that some ambulance services have taken to training crews specially for both general emergency work and service in ambulances equipped to deal with the victims of heart attack. At the same time, increasing numbers of general practitioners and some hospital doctors have been taking part in the care of emergency cases on the spot, particularly after road accidents.

Special emergency services

The purpose of these services is to try to reduce the mortality and morbidity of road accidents, in particular by providing a higher standard of care and equipment and in some cases by accelerating the arrival of such a service at the place of accident. The initiative in setting up such organizations has come from doctors, who have recognized the importance of co-ordinating the activities of the police and the fire and ambulance services as well as contributing their own.

The course of events is usually for the police to receive first news of an accident and then to notify the other emergency services. The fire service is used as much for its rescue equipment as for its ability to prevent or quench fires. The nearest participating doctor is also notified and he sets off in his own vehicle with his emergency kit. Whichever organization arrives first does what it can until the others arrive and can assume their proper responsibilities. This can result in there being a doctor on the spot before anyone else; on other occasions the ambulance may be ready to leave for hospital before the doctor has arrived. If this is the case the ambulance is not required to await the arrival of the doctor unless its crew particularly feel the need for medical advice or assistance.

A big advantage of this scheme is that by calling the doctor in all cases treatment for the patient may be accelerated. This advantage has to be set against the waste of medical time in many cases. In this connection, it should be pointed out that the essence of any emergency service is the ability to act at a moment's notice, in consequence of which much of its time is spent waiting.

Another system is to have a doctor, or a medical team, available to answer calls by one or other of emergency services when they feel the need for medical assistance.

Arrangements like these have a dramatic appeal and a measure of the enthusiasm they engender is the fact that about 1,300 doctors taking part in such schemes have been financed by private funds amounting to as much as several hundred pounds each when radio transmitters and receivers are carried. Basic equipment such as splints, dressings, resuscitation apparatus, protective clothing and warning signs costs about £100.

The role of the doctor

Doctors can be regarded as having two roles. Firstly to be first on the scene and secondly to provide a standard of care above that of the other emergency services. These may be jointly expressed as trying to prevent preventable deaths and morbidity. There has been more or less enthusiastic advocacy of medical participation in road-side care but with more assertion than evidence that it saves many lives or much morbidity. It has been inferred that if at necropsy 20 per cent or more of persons dying shortly after accidents are found to have blood, vomitus or the like in the respiratory tract it should be possible to save this proportion of deaths after accidents, particularly on the roads. Such inference is fallacious because about half the deaths occur in hospital and also because it is not unusual for a dying person to regurgitate and inhale gastric contents, which may accelerate but does not cause his death.

Several surveys have suggested that the number of preventable deaths is less than 5 per cent of those caused by road accidents and one survey indicates that there are probably more preventable deaths after patients reach hospital than before.

With such conflicting opinions and evidence it is obviously desirable that there should be a sound basis for deciding the value of doctors at the place of accident.

Advanced training in the ambulance service

Just as medical enthusiasm has taken doctors out to accidents, so has it sought to improve the skills of ambulance crews. This is nothing new; in Hungary, for example, 'medical officers' (who are not doctors) are trained in resuscitation by intravenous infusion and intubation of the trachea and other methods that will enable them to work in active co-operation with doctors, or independently if necessary.

Britain has at least two services that are offering advanced training. In Gloucestershire crews are trained in hospitals, where they are in effect part of the staff, and to which they return from time to time for refresher courses. In Brighton, crews have been trained in the diagnosis and treatment of heart attacks, using electrocardiography and electrical defibrillation as well as intravenous infusion and endotracheal intubation. Such training is practicable and it has aroused great interest and enthusiasm so it may be asked why advanced training is not now recommended for the country as a whole.

Evaluation of advanced training

One answer is that enthusiasm and satisfaction are not in themselves sufficient justification for a striking change in policy. The questions that need to be answered are:

Is there a need for advanced training for ambulance crews, and for the participation of doctors in similar emergency work? In other words, how many lives can be saved by these measures and is there clear evidence that morbidity is reduced?

Is there reason to think that special training is more effective than good First Aid or 'Ambulance Aid' whithin the first hour or so of a serious accident?

If advanced training is worth while, is there need for it throughout the country? If not, where and to whom should it be made available? A study of fatal road accidents in and around Birmingham provided no encouragement for advocates of advanced training for urban accidents but suggested that it might save some lives in the cases of rural accidents. Practical experience of a mobile surgical team in Birmingham led to its being abandoned on the grounds of great expense to very little purpose. In contrast to this, however, experience in other parts of the country has been more favourable towards flying squads despatched from hospitals to deal with the victims of serious accidents and enthusiasm has continued to flourish because there are few facts upon which convincing opposition can be based. There is no doubt that lives have been saved and for the enthusiast that is enough, whereas the state understandably requires convincing evidence that it should assume financial responsibility for what has so far been paid for by subscription and private generosity.

Evaluation of the work of doctors and ambulance crews with special training is most likely to be achieved by prompt and careful examination of their written and verbal reports by a suitably experienced doctor who will have seen the patient in hospital and will therefore be in a position to compare 'outdoor' diagnoses with those that are finally accepted, and to decide the need for and the efficacy of whatever advanced and medical aid has been provided.

The fact that a person is resuscitated at the place of accident and reaches hospital alive is no justification for the service responsible if the patient then dies from irremediable injuries, nor again if it turns out that the patient's injuries were less severe than was at first thought to be the case and that elaborate treatment was unnecessary. What is convincing is that a person choking to death is turned on his side and makes a complete recovery. These are important matters and need careful study. Such a study should be carried out in urban and in rural areas and particularly in areas in which ambulances might take half an hour to reach the patient and perhaps as long again to carry him to hospital; furthermore it should be planned to compare the work of doctors, specially trained ambulance crews and those with the ordinary proficiency certificate. Such facts as have so far been published suggest that the following policy is reasonable at present.

In a large town or city, the standard training of the ambulance service is sufficient but the hospital service should provide a medical team for resuscitation of trapped and severely injured persons.

In the country, particularly where the population is scattered and hospitals are widely separated medical participation should be encouraged, if for no other reason than to get knowledgeable help to casualties as soon as possible. Ambulance crews in such areas should receive special training to enable them to deal more effectively with the hazards that beset patients increasingly as their journeys to hsopital become longer.

It seems reasonable to require that if the state is to support these ventures it should be provided with the means of appraising them. As evidence of the relative values of the different participants and their standards of training and equipment become available it may be possible to dispose the necessary skills more economically.

It will be recognized that the foregoing remarks apply mostly to Great Britain and that the value of highly organized services that include doctors and police and military helicopters has been accepted in Vietnam, the United States and Australia, in conditions that bear little resemblance to those in Britain. The essential requirement in such elaborate schemes is good communication, which means using an existing service that can readily be made available at all times.

Insurance

An important consideration in all potentially hazardous work is that those taking part should be suitably insured against death or disablement, which are by no means negligible hazards after accidents on express roads.

TRANSPORT

Conveyance by road

A long-recurring complaint is that the ill and hurt are delivered to hospital in what are in effect merely disguised, if well equipped, delivery vans. There is no doubt that medical advances have been made in the last 70 or 80 years (*Figures 12.2, 12.3, 12.4*), but whatever the patient has gained in speed of conveyance has not been matched by comfort.

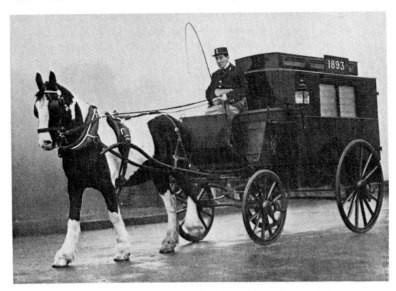

Figure 12.2. An ambulance of the Metropolitan Asylums' Board
(By courtesy of the London Ambulance Service)

What is required

A great deal of thought and practical effort has been devoted to the specification and design of ambulances and the essentials include the following.

A low floor to facilitate loading.
A comfortable working height for the crew.
Central fittings for the stretcher so that the attendant has easy access to the patient from all sides.
Equipment so placed that in an emergency the patient's attendant can reach what he needs without leaving the head of the patient.
An equable internal temperature in both hot and cold weather.
Adequate lighting inside.
Insulation against undue noise.
A comfortable ride.

It is in the last respect that good intentions have been most frustrated by practical difficulties.

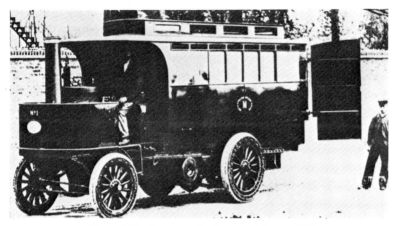

Figure 12.3. Thornycroft steam ambulance, 1902
(By courtesy of the London Ambulance Service)

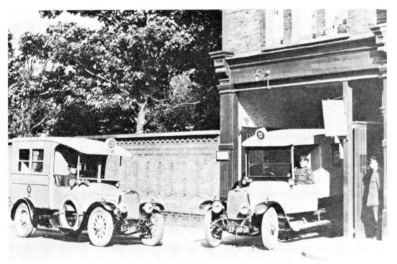

Figure 12.4. Southwestern (later Brixton) ambulance station, 1923
(By courtesy of the London Ambulance Service)

Cost

The British market does not require more than about 500 new ambulances a year and most of these are not used only for carrying seriously injured persons. The need for economy obliges ambulance services to use many of their vehicles for the carriage of either one or two stretcher patients or up to 10 seated persons. The mechanical characteristics of a vehicle that is suitable for the latter purpose are inappropriate for the former. Even with a much larger market, the cost of designing and building a special vehicle is deterrent, if not prohibitive. The solution that would be most likely to be accepted would be to design a vehicle that would make use of the most suitable mass-produced parts. Even so, there is much that needs to be known.

Ignorance

For all the money and effort that have been spent on comfort in conveyances they have been concerned mostly with seated passengers who can see something of where they are going. A patient on a stretcher in an ambulance has neither warning of change in the vehicle's speed or direction, nor of changes in the smoothness of the road, nor means of bracing himself against them.

A possible alternative is to concentrate on building a stretcher that will protect the patient from the undesirable accelerations of an ordinary commercial vehicle. One such suspension has in fact been made but it had the unfortunate effect of replacing painful jolts by nauseating swaying but there is reason to think that this disadvantage has been overcome by a new stretcher of Dutch origin.

In spite of the practical difficulties of studying the reactions of sick and injured persons to different sorts of ambulance journeys modern techniques of measuring and recording phsyiological, and perhaps pathological, responses to changes in the environment give reason to hope that useful information will become available within the next few years. The extent to which this information might be expressed in the design of better ambulances remains to be seen.

Conveyance by air

Air ambulances of one sort or another have been in use for many years, ranging in their purpose from the urgent conveyance of one person to the planned movement of large numbers of casualties caused by enemy action or natural disaster.

Some countries include aircraft in their ambulance service and in Britain the Order of St John has its Air Wing, which does not confine its activities to the carriage of patients.

Helicopters

Such use of air transport has become well enough established not to occasion much comment or debate but the use of helicopters has introduced a note of eagerness and of enthusiasm for its special characteristics. It is tempting to suppose that helicopters can be summoned almost as easily as taxicabs and that they will then whisk the patient away from an otherwise inaccessible position and convey him smoothly and swiftly to wherever his condition requires. The facts, at least in Britain, do not support these suppositions.

The largest number of helicopters in Britain belongs to the Army Air Corps but many of those at present in use will accommodate one patient on a stretcher, which has to be a special one because standard stretchers are too big. However, larger machines are becoming available.

The other two Services provide helicopters for rescue at sea. Their bases are all on or near the coast and they are widely separated. The machines are available for civilian use if they are not required by the Services.

Many hours may elapse between the request for a helicopter and its arrival to collect the patient. A survey of the use of helicopters in Britain showed that if travelling time were regarded as the interval between calling for a helicopter and the arrival of the patient at his destination, the average speed of travel was 64 km per hour (40 miles per hour). There is thus no possibility of using these machines to swoop down, for example, within minutes of a crash on an express road.

Few civilian firms provide helicopters and they have even more widely separated bases than the Services. Nevertheless, when machines are in regular use, supplying drilling platforms in the North Sea, for example, they can serve medical purposes at relatively less cost.

Generally speaking, the use of helicopters falls under one of the following headings.

Courtesy

Civilian use of Service helicopters in Britain is a courtesy. The objectives include rescue from inaccessible places, a smooth and fairly swift journey of 80 km (50 miles) or more, particularly when this can be planned.

Operational necessity

In war, cost is a less important consideration than it is in peace and it is often possible to know when and where casualties will occur and in roughly what numbers. The success of the US Army's use of helicopters in Vietnam owed much to scientific and technical excellence and enthusiasm and even more to complete command of the air. The success achieved there has given great impetus to civilian medical enthusiasts.

Policy

The state of Maryland has set a remarkable standard by using the helicopters and the communications system of its state police as a basis for a state-wide organization to carry the sick and injured as swiftly as possible to special emergency units, to provide skilled care on the way, to take care to where it will be required and to carry organs that are to be transported. By making use (which amounts to about 10 per cent of the 2,000 or so hours flown each year) of an existing fleet of helicopters the medical authorities have saved themselves a great deal of money. The excellence of such a service, and a similar one in Germany, depends upon the fact that a suitable organization is already in existence and can make itself available for another purpose. These conditions do not exist in Britain.

Other forms of conveyance

Rail

The hospital train is useful in war but the design of modern coaching stock makes it impossible for a stretcher patient to travel in a passenger coach; he has to be content with the guard's van.

Sea

Any hospital ships in the future will be the result of modifying a passenger vessel but the commando carriers of the Royal Navy provide comprehensive medical facilities for the fighting men they carry. On a much smaller scale are the life-boats and in particular, the specially equipped motor launch, 'Flying Christine', that the energy and initiative of Mr Blanchford, CStJ, has made available round the coasts of Guernsey. In accidents at sea the prime consideration is getting the casualty to a place of safety. Treatment on the way may be restricted to lashing him firmly and safely in place. Hovercraft have characteristics that give them a special place among methods of transport but steadiness and quietness are not among them and it is only the largest craft that can travel over fairly rough water or uneven ground.

Dangerous pastimes

Pot-holing and mountain-climbing pose special problems of rescue, conveyance and protection against cold, wet and impact and falling

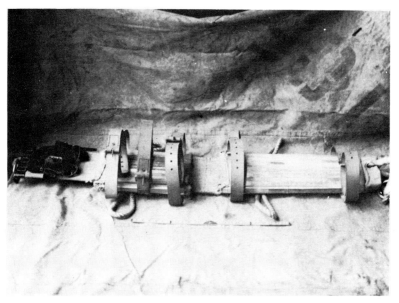

Figure 12.5. Neil Robertson's stretcher

objects while in transit; and their rescue services have devised or adapted suitable splints and stretchers (*Figures 12.5–12.9*).

COMMUNICATIONS

The foundation of any emergency service is the ability to make the occurrence of an emergency known without delay to whichever persons and organizations have a contribution to make in dealing with it.

Radio

In spite of the reluctance of the authorities to increase the load of radio facilities there has been a useful co-ordination of the networks of the different services and a readiness to share facilities in some cases.

Apart from the convenience of being able at any time to ascertain and control the activities of individual persons and component units of an emergency service, radio has allowed ambulance crews in difficulties

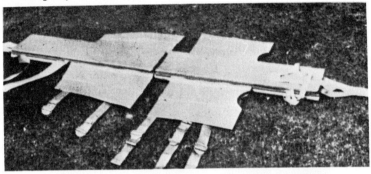

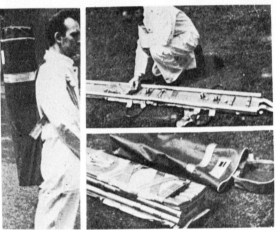

Figure 12.6. Paraguard stretcher, which is lighter, less cumbersome and more durable than Neil Robertson's and can be carried on the back
(By courtesy of Vicker's Medical)

to seek advice of doctors in hospital and to offer detailed warning of what type of casualties they are about to take to the hospital.

Telemetry

Another technique that has been used is to transmit to a doctor in hospital patients' electrocardiograms and records of blood pressure and other vital processes so that he can advise the crew. This carries the difficulties of using the equipment in unfavourable conditions and the danger that the attendant will be more attentive to the apparatus than to the patient. Advanced training is more likely, in the long run, to provide comparable safeguards with fewer disadvantages.

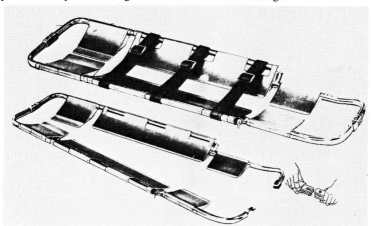

Figure 12.7. Scoop stretcher, which can be slipped under a patient without lifting him. The two parts can be parted at one or both ends, which can facilitate the use of this stretcher. Note the locking device and the retaining strips
(By courtesy of F. W. Equipment Co Ltd)

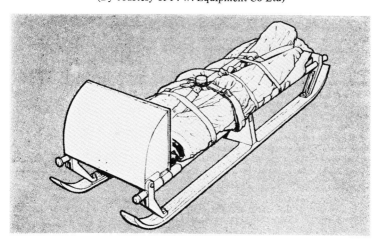

Figure 12.8. The Duff stretcher, which can be used on ice and snow and offers protection for the patient's head. Note the quick-release box on the retaining harness
(By courtesy of Her Majesty's Stationary Office, from RAF Handbook on Mountain Rescue)

In a number of ways the future offers interesting and even exciting prospects in the earliest stages of the care of the seriously ill and hurt. When so much is technically possible and when, for some purposes,

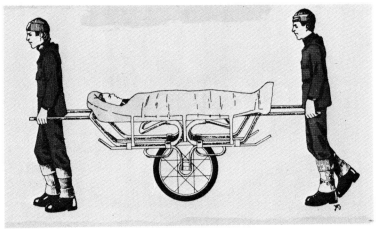

Figure 12.9. The MacInnes stretcher has extending handles, yokes, side grips, ski runners and a detachable wheel
(By courtesy of Update Publications)

there is no counting of cost it is important that an honest attempt should be made to evaluate developments so they can be realized as useful advances rather than expensive changes.

FURTHER READING

BASIC FIRST AID

First Aid (1972). London; St John Ambulance Association and Brigade
Miles, S. (1970). *Ballière's Handbook of First Aid.* London; Ballière, Tindall
— and Roylance, P. J. (1970). *Teaching First Aid.* London; Ballière, Tindall
Occupational First Aid (1973). London; St. John Ambulance Assocation and Brigade
Taylor, Lord (1974). *First Aid in the Factory.* London; Longman

ADVANCED FIRST AID

Gardner, A. W. and Roylance, P. J. (1967). *New Essential First Aid.* London; Pan Books
— and — (1969). *New Advanced First Aid.* London; Butterworths
Mountain Rescue (1968). London; HMSO
Playfair, A. S. (1973). *Modern First Aid.* Middx.; Hamlyn
Snook, R. (1974). *Medical Aid at Accidents.* Update Publications

TRAINING OF AMBULANCE CREWS

Ministry of Health Circular 30/51 (1951). *'Supplementary training of ambulance staff.'* London; HMSO
Morris, S. C. (1970). *A Complete Handbook for Professional Ambulance Personnel.* Bristol; John Wright & Sons
Report by Gloucestershire Ambulance Service on Advanced Ambulance Training (1974). *'Mobile resuscitation units.'*
Report by the Working Party on Ambulance Training (1966). London; HMSO
White, N. M., Parker, W. S., Binning, R. A., Kimber, E. R., Ead, H. W. and Chamberlain, D. A. (1973). 'Mobile coronary care provided by ambulance personnel.' *Br. med. J.* 3, 618

DESIGN AND EQUIPMENT OF AMBULANCES

Medical Commission on Accident Prevention (1969). International seminar on design criteria for the emergency ambulance
Report by the Working Party on Ambulance Equipment (1967). London; HMSO

271

ROAD ACCIDENTS AND MEDICAL AID

Department of Transportation and Environmental Planning; the University of Birmingham (1969). 'Causes and effects of road accidents.'

Mackay, G. M. (1969). 'Some features of traffic accidents.' *Br. Med. J.* **4,** 799

Pacy, H. (1971). *Road Accidents–Medical Aid.* Edinburgh; Livingstone

INDEX